CATHERINE SIENNA

HERBAL REMEDIES
The How and Why

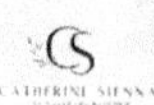

First edition

*This book was professionally typeset on
Reedsy. Find out more at reedsy.com*

CONTENTS

CHAPTER 1
INTRODUCTION TO HERBAL REMEDIES

CHAPTER 5 UNDERSTANDING PLANT IDENTIFICATION AND HARVESTING

1 CHAPTER

Introduction to Herbal Remedies

In a world dominated by modern medicine, the use of herbal remedies may seem like a thing of the past. However, the healing power of plants has been recognized and utilized for centuries in different cultures around the world. Herbal remedies, also known as herbal medicine or botanical medicine, involve the use of various plant parts, such as leaves, flowers, roots, and bark, to promote health and well-being (Weltz, et al. 2018).

The concept of herbal medicine is deeply rooted in human history and stems from ancient civilizations' observations and interactions with nature. Throughout time, traditional healers and herbalists accumulated knowledge about the medicinal properties of plants through trial and error passed down through generations. They carefully studied and identified plant species based on their distinct characteristics, understanding that different parts of the plant can possess different therapeutic properties (Schwab, et al. 2020).

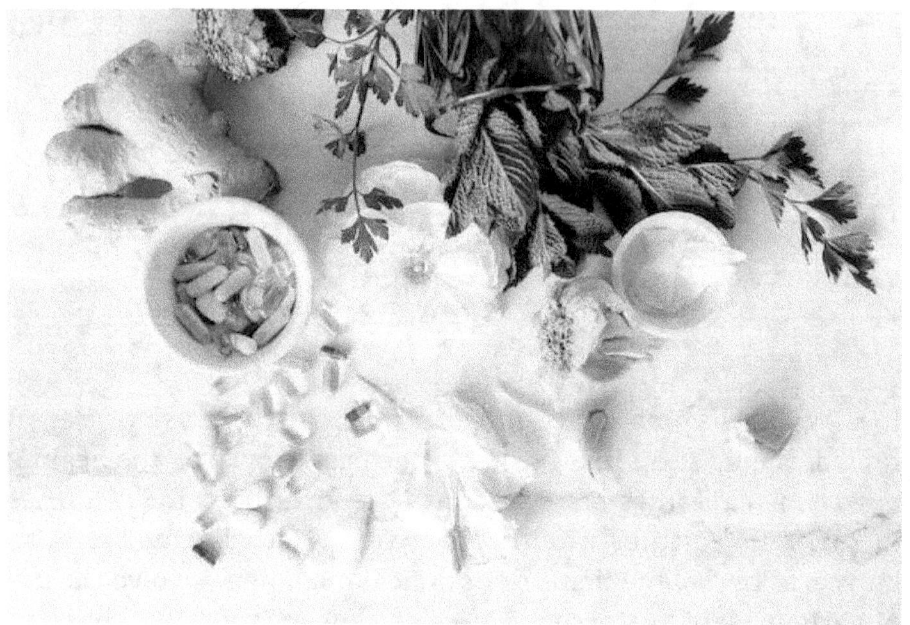

Herbal medicine is a holistic approach to health, focusing on addressing the root cause of ailments rather than just alleviating specific symptoms. It acknowledges the interconnections of various bodily systems, emphasizing the importance of overall well-being. The body is viewed as a complex and integrated ecosystem, where achieving harmony is essential for optimal health (Weltz, et al. 2018). By supporting the body's innate healing mechanisms, herbal remedies help restore balance and promote long-term vitality.

One of the advantages of herbal remedies lies in their rich diversity and adaptability. Plants with medicinal properties can be found in every corner of the world, flourishing in different environments, and adapting to specific conditions. Traditional healers and indigenous communities have developed deep relationships with these plants, recognizing their unique properties and understanding how to extract their healing potential. They have passed down this knowledge through oral traditions, sharing their remedies and techniques across generations.

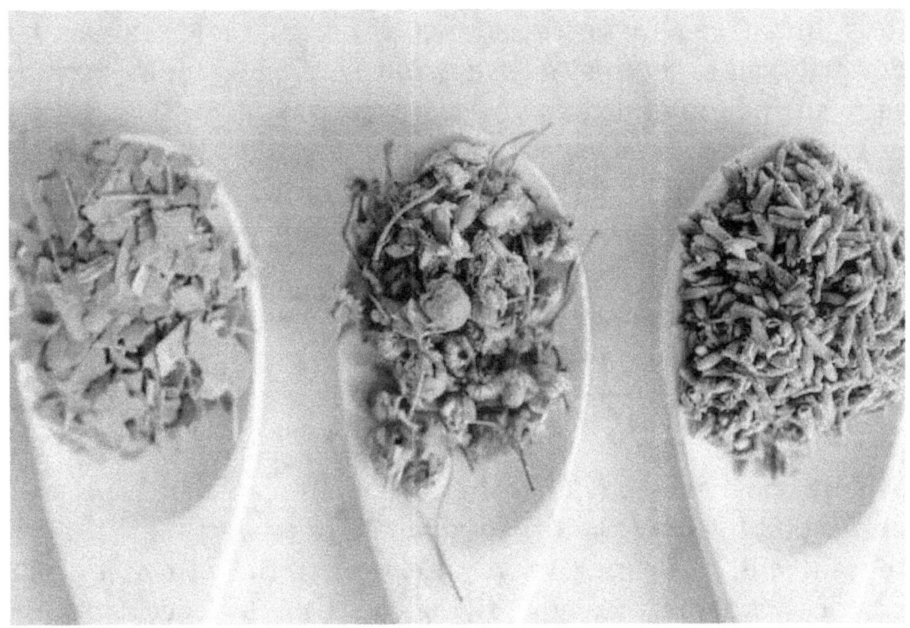

The process of harnessing the healing potential of plants involves various techniques that have been refined over time. Traditional healers carefully consider factors such as the environment and season in which the plant grows, as well as the methods of cultivation, harvesting, and preparation that optimize the plant's medicinal qualities. They understand that the potency and effectiveness of herbal remedies depend on these factors and adjust their approach accordingly.

Preparation methods for herbal remedies can vary widely and may include the use of teas, tinctures, poultices, infusions, capsules, or topical applications. Each method facilitates the extraction and concentration of active plant compounds, making them more readily available for absorption by the body. Moreover, the choice of preparation method can be influenced by the plant's specific properties and the desired outcome. For example, certain plants may be more effective when ingested, while others may have a stronger impact when applied topically.

It is important to note that while herbal remedies can be powerful allies in maintaining and improving one's health, they are not intended to replace professional medical advice or treatment. It is always advisable to consult with a qualified healthcare practitioner before incorporating herbal remedies into your routine, especially if you have an existing medical condition or are taking prescribed medications. They can effectively guide you in utilizing herbal remedies safely and ensuring their compatibility with your specific health needs.

In this book, we will embark on a comprehensive journey into the fascinating world of herbal remedies. We will explore the intricate relationships between plants and humans, understanding how plants have adapted to provide remedies for the ailments we face. We will delve into the principles and practices of herbal medicine, giving you the knowledge and tools to engage with natural remedies confidently.

Each chapter will focus on specific areas of health, such as digestion, sleep, energy, and immune support, and provide a comprehensive guide to the herbs most commonly used for those purposes. We will uncover the characteristics, properties, and benefits of individual herbs, enabling you to make informed choices and select appropriate remedies for your unique well-being.

As we navigate through the pages of this book, we encourage you to cultivate a deep appreciation for nature's wisdom and recognize the profound relationship between humans and plants. By embracing herbal remedies, you have the opportunity to tap into the rich heritage of our ancestors, connecting with ancient traditions while embracing the advancements of modern science.

Together, let us unlock the remarkable healing potential of nature's bounty and empower ourselves with knowledge and understanding of herbal remedies. May our journey lead to improved well-being, balance, and harmony.

CHAPTER 2
History and Evolution of Herbal Medicine

Throughout history, humans have relied on the healing power of plants for their medicinal needs. Herbal medicine, also known as botanical medicine or herbalism, has been practiced by different cultures around the world for thousands of years. This chapter aims to explore the fascinating history and evolution of herbal medicine, shedding light on its origins and its journey to become one of the most widely used forms of healthcare.

The roots of herbal medicine can be traced back to ancient civilizations, including those of the Egyptians, Greeks, Chinese, and Indians. These cultures recognized the therapeutic properties of various plants and documented their use in treating a wide range of ailments. From the famous Egyptian Ebers Papyrus to the Indian Ayurvedic texts and the Chinese Materia Medica, these ancient writings provide valuable insights into the medicinal plants and herbal remedies of their time.

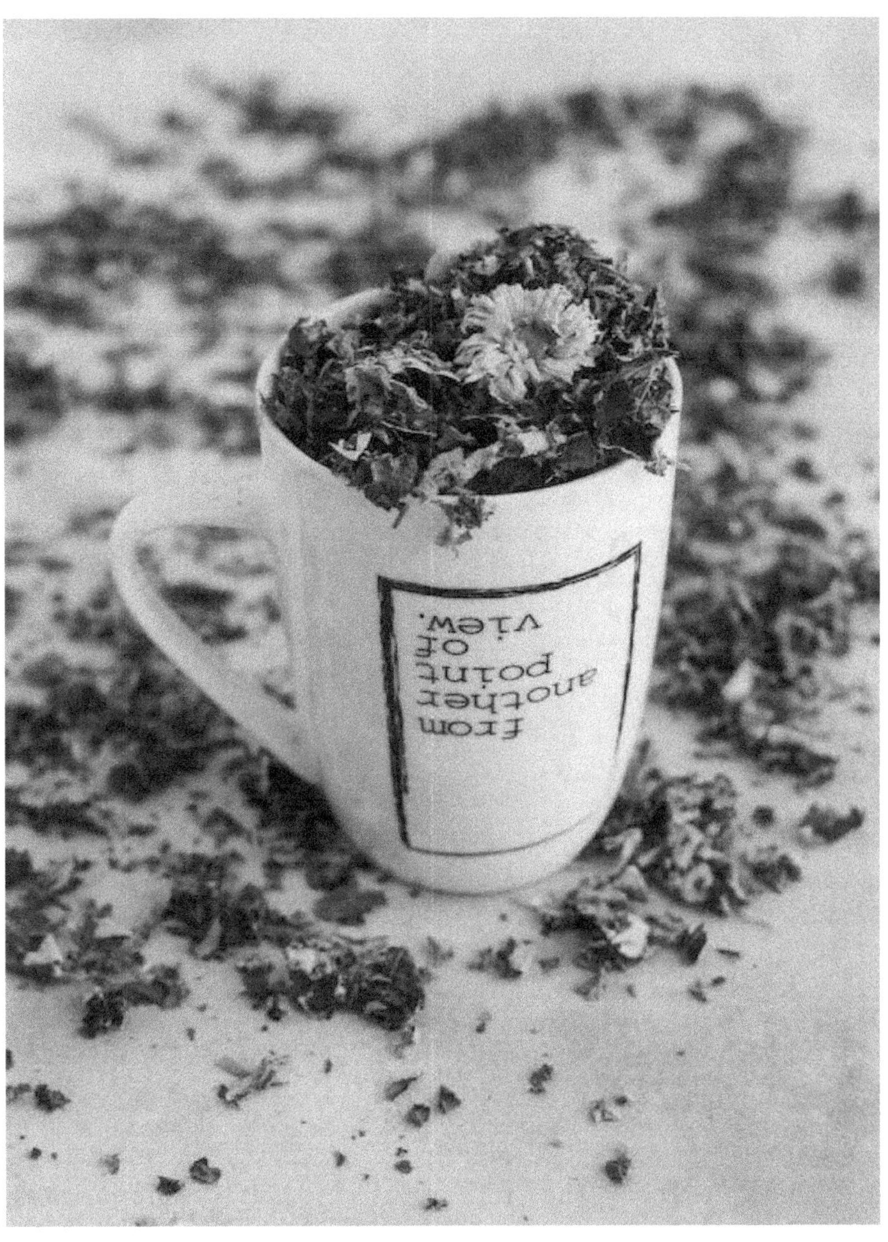
from
another
of
view.

The Ancient Egyptians were known for their advanced knowledge of herbal medicine, using plants like aloe vera, myrrh, and frankincense for healing purposes. They believed that these plants possessed both physical and spiritual healing properties, often incorporating them into religious rituals and ceremonies. The Ebers Papyrus, dating back to around 1550 BCE, contains information about over 850 herbal remedies, including opium poppy for pain relief and garlic for its antiseptic properties.

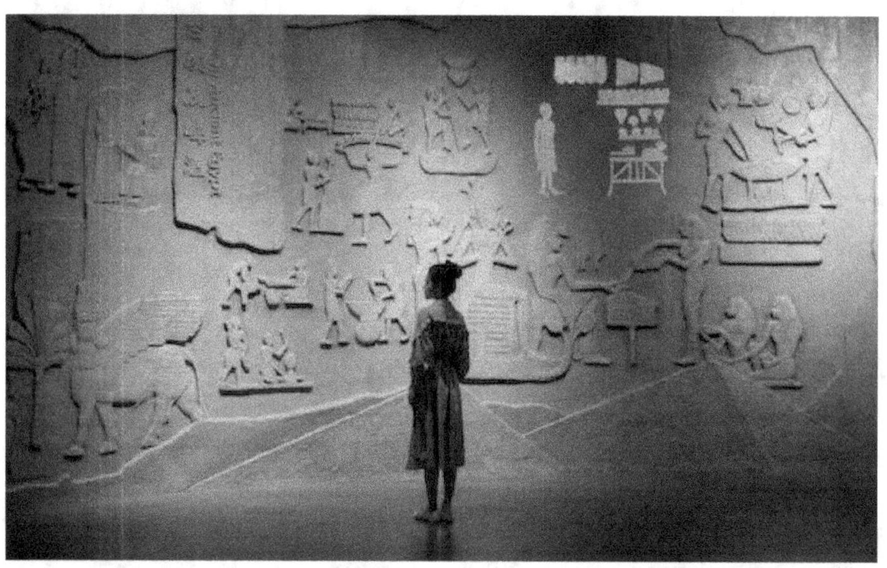

In ancient Greece, the father of medicine, Hippocrates, emphasized the importance of using plants as medicine. He believed in the concept of holistic healing and developed the theory of the four humors, which suggested that imbalances in the body's fluids could lead to illness. Herbal remedies, such as chamomile, garlic, and peppermint, were commonly prescribed by Greek physicians. The writings of Hippocrates and his followers, known as the Hippocratic Corpus, include detailed descriptions of various herbs, their properties, and their uses in treating different diseases.

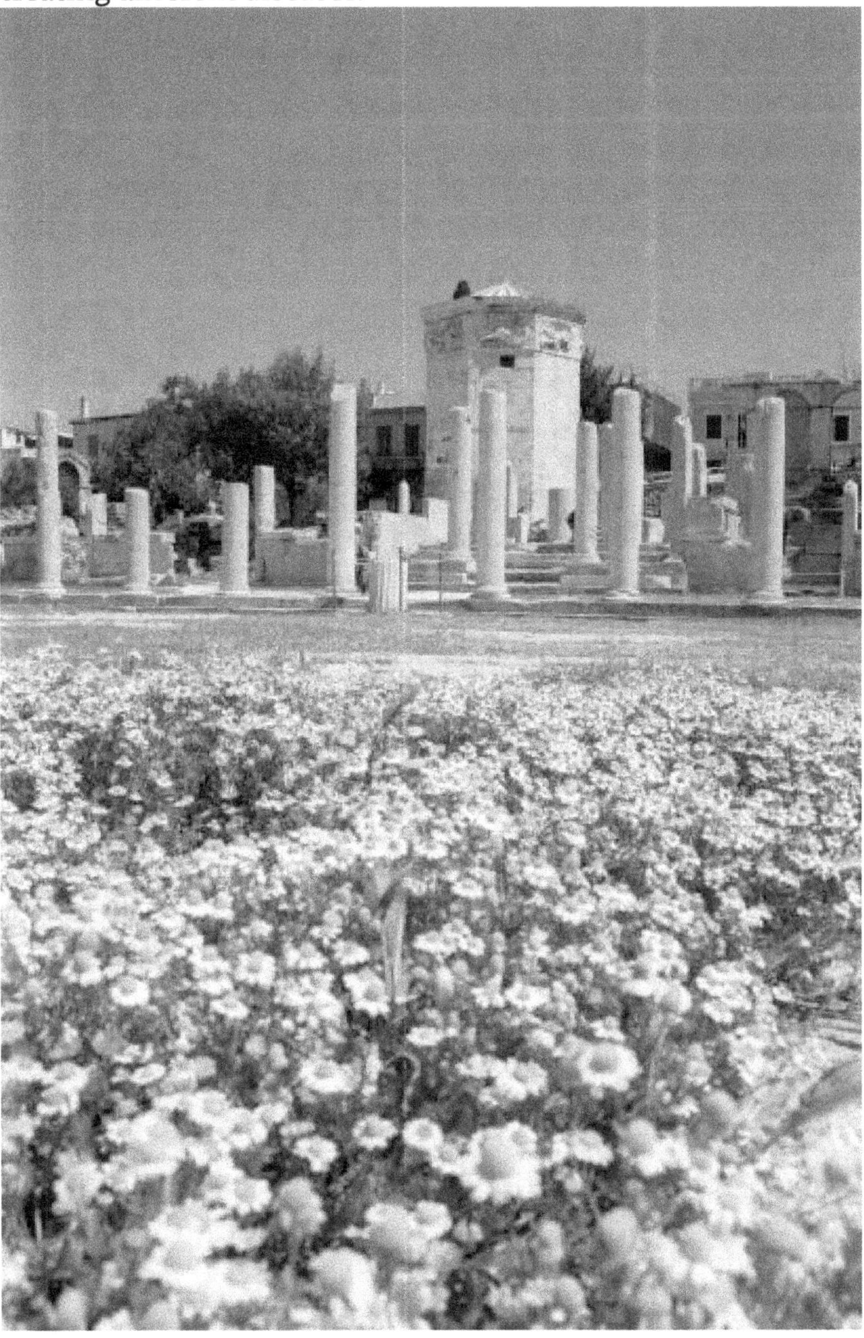

In traditional Chinese medicine (TCM), the understanding of herbal medicine is deeply rooted in the concept of Qi (pronounced chee) or life force energy. Chinese herbalists formulate remedies using a combination of herbs tailored to each individual's unique constitution. Ginseng, ginger, and licorice are some of the well-known herbs used in TCM to restore balance and promote health. The ancient Chinese medical text, the Yellow Emperor's Inner Canon (Huangdi Neijing), provides a comprehensive understanding of Chinese herbal medicine, including the principles of diagnosis and treatment.

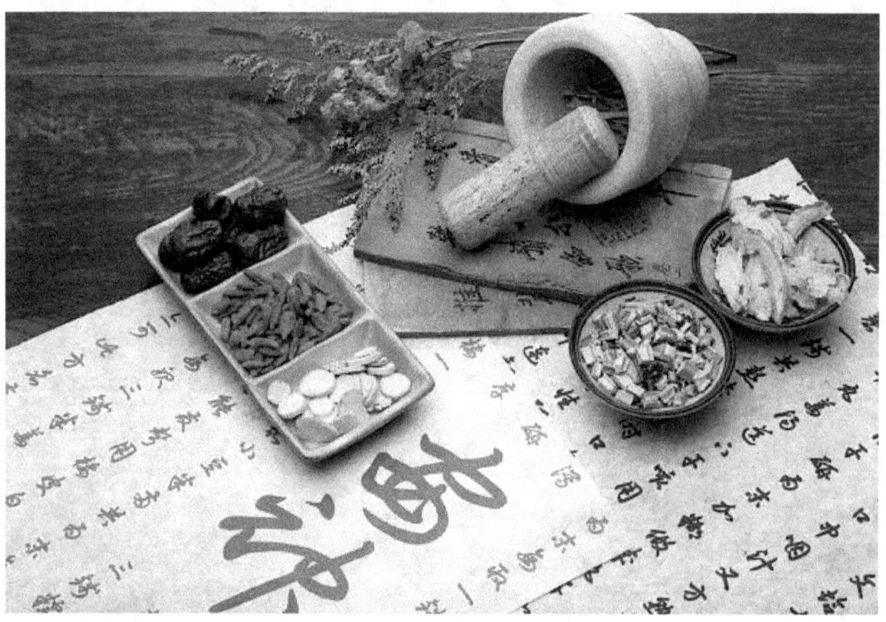

Similarly, Ayurveda, the traditional medicine system of India, has a long history of using herbal remedies. Ayurvedic texts, such as Charaka Samhita and Sushruta Samhita, describe the use of plants like turmeric, neem, and ashwagandha for their medicinal properties. Ayurvedic practitioners focus on maintaining balance between the body, mind, and spirit to achieve optimal health. They consider factors such as individual constitution (dosha), seasons, and lifestyle when prescribing herbal remedies.

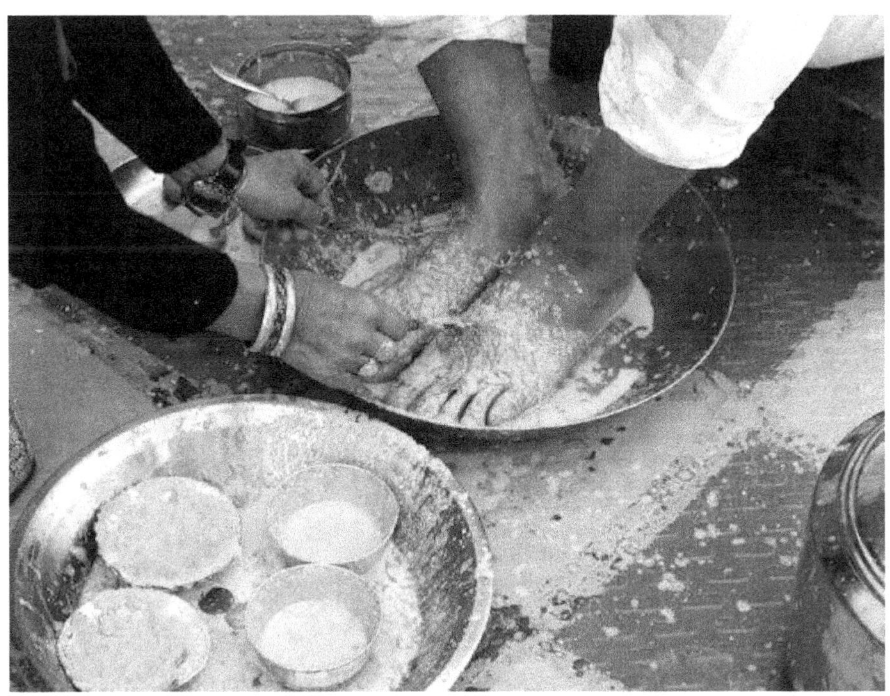

As civilization advanced, herbal medicine continued to evolve. The Renaissance period witnessed a resurgence of interest in botanical medicine as explorers traveled the world, discovering new plants with medicinal properties. The development of modern pharmacology and the isolation of active chemical compoundsfromplantsinthe19thcenturyledtotheproduction of standardized herbal medicines. This era also saw the emergence of influential herbalists and botanists, such as Nicholas Culpeper and Samuel Thomson, who documented the uses of various herbs and their preparations.

Today, herbal medicine remains an integral part of healthcare in many cultures, including traditional systems of medicine like TCM and Ayurveda (Schwab, et al. 2023). Furthermore, there has been a growing interest in herbal medicine in Western societies, as people seek natural alternatives to conventional treatments.

Scientific research continues to explore the medicinal properties of plants, validating their traditional uses and uncovering new therapeutic potentials.

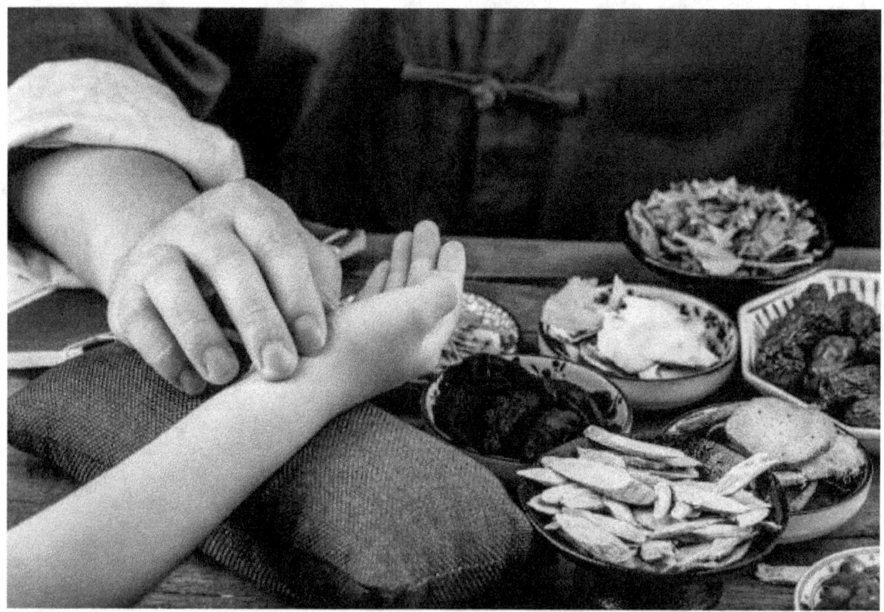

The history and evolution of herbal medicine reflect the enduring relationship between humans and the botanical world. From ancient civilizations to modern times, the quest for natural healing has driven the exploration and utilization of plants for their medicinal benefits. It is important to note that while herbal medicine has a long history of traditional use, not all herbal remedies are safe or effective. Some herbs can interact with medications or have adverse effects, underscoring the importance of consulting with qualified healthcare professionals and utilizing evidence-based information.

In recent years, there has been an increased emphasis on evidence-based herbal medicine. This approach combines traditional knowledge with scientific research to validate the efficacy and safety of herbal remedies. Researchers conduct studies to understand the active compounds present in medicinal plants, their mechanisms of action, and potential interactions with other medications. The aim is to develop standardized herbal preparations and guidelines for their use, ensuring quality control and consistent dosing.

The rise of herbal medicine has also given birth to various professional organizations and regulatory bodies that promote education, training, and ethical practice. These institutions work towards establishing professional standards, ensuring the safe and effective use of herbal remedies. Integrative medicine, which combines conventional medicine with complementary therapies, including herbal medicine, is gaining recognition and acceptance in healthcare systems worldwide.

By studying the history and evolution of herbal medicine, we can appreciate not only the traditional wisdom but also the ongoing research and innovation in this field. The synergy between traditional knowledge and scientific advancements holds great potential for expanding therapeutic options available to individuals seeking holistic and natural approaches to healthcare.

Herbal medicine has a rich and diverse history that spans across cultures and centuries. From ancient civilizations to modern times, the healing power of plants has been valued and utilized. The continued exploration, research, and integration of herbal medicine into healthcare systems worldwide are a testament to its enduring relevance and potential for enhancing health and well-being. It is important to approach herbal medicine with scientific rigor, ensuring safety, efficacy, and informed decision-making for the benefit of individuals seeking alternative healthcare options.

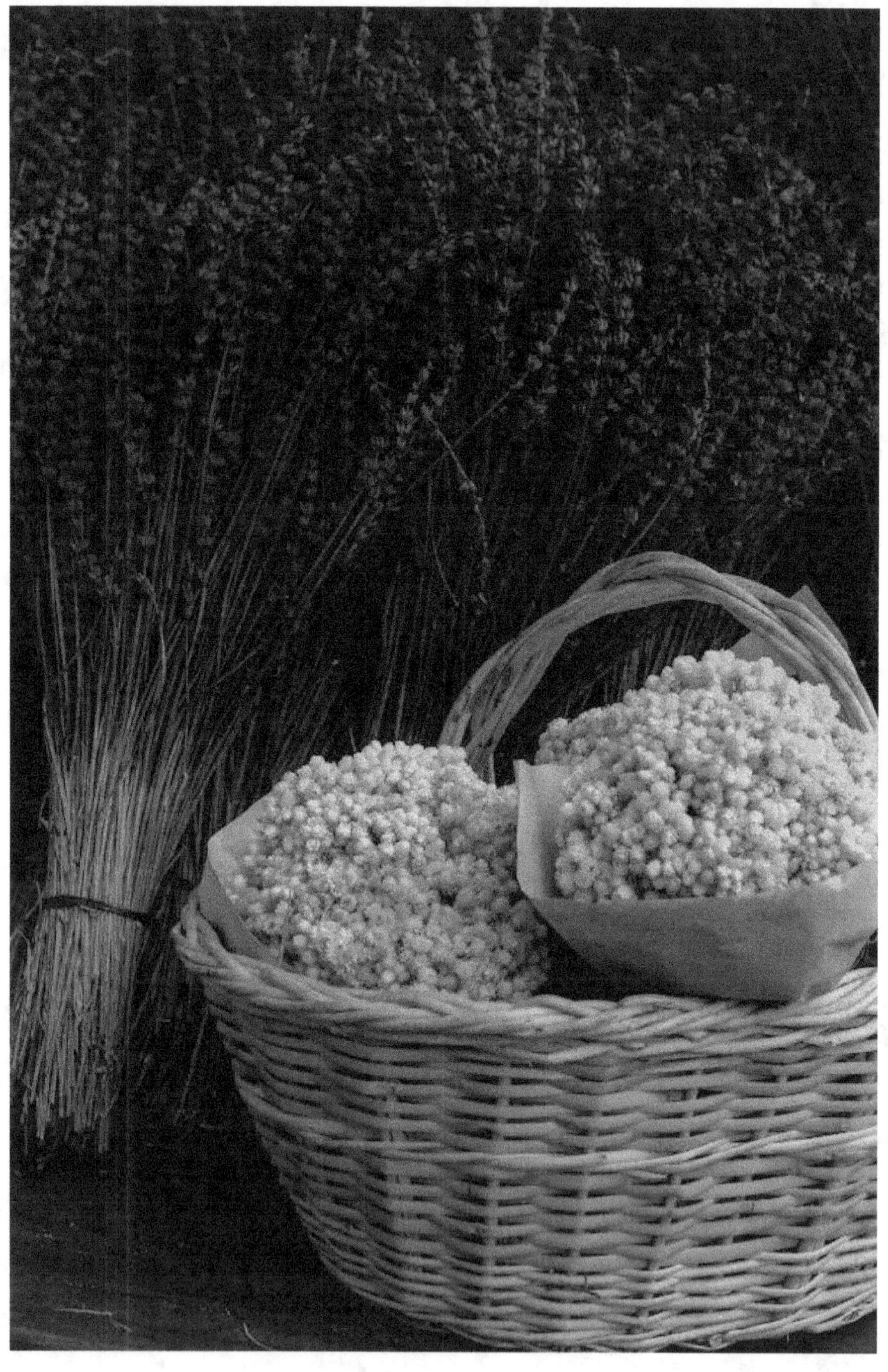

CHAPTER 3
Principles of Herbal Medicine

Herbal medicine, also known as herbalism or phytotherapy, has been practiced for centuries and is rooted in the belief that plants possess medicinal properties that can promote healing and wellness in the human body. Understanding the core principles of herbal medicine is essential for anyone interested in harnessing the power of plants for their health and well-being. These principles guide herbalists in their practice, ensuring safe and effective treatments while embracing the holistic nature of human health.

1. **Holistic Approach:**

Herbal medicine takes a holistic approach to health, recognizing the interconnections of the mind, body, and spirit. It acknowledges that imbalances or diseases in one aspect of a person can affect other areas as well. Rather than simply addressing the symptoms, herbal medicine aims to identify and treat the root causes of illness, considering both physical and emotional aspects of a person's well-being. By restoring overall harmony, herbal medicine seeks to promote long-lasting wellness.

2. **Individualized Treatment:**

Herbal medicine acknowledges the uniqueness of each individual and tailor's treatments based on their specific needs. Herbalists consider an individual's constitution, genetic makeup, health history, emotional well-being, and environmental factors when determining the appropriate herbs and remedies. By customizing treatment plans, herbalists aim to address the specific imbalances or conditions of each person, supporting their journey toward optimal health.

3. **Plant Identification:**

An essential skill in herbal medicine is the proper identification of medicinal plants. This involves learning to recognize different species and varieties of plants, understanding their botanical characteristics, and being able to differentiate between medicinal plants and their look-alike. Knowledge of plant families, growth habits, habitat preferences, and therapeutic actions ensure the safe and effective use of herbal remedies. Herbalists also understand the importance of sustainable wildcrafting practices and ethical sourcing of herbal materials.

4. **Active Constituents:**

Herbal medicine recognizes that plants contain numerous active constituents that contribute to their therapeutic properties. These constituents include alkaloids, flavonoids, glycosides, phenols, terpenes, and essential oils, among others. Understanding the constituents present in each herb helps determine their specific actions in the body, such as analgesic, anti-inflammatory, antimicrobial, or adaptogenic effects. With this knowledge, herbalists can select appropriate herbs for individual health conditions, considering their specific biochemical interactions.

5. **Traditional Wisdom and Scientific Evidence:**

Herbal medicine combines traditional knowledge and wisdom with modern scientific research. It values the wisdom passed down through generations of herbalists, folk healers, and indigenous cultures, as well as the insights gained from contemporary evidence-based studies. This integration bridges the gap between ancient wisdom and modern scientific discoveries, providing a comprehensive understanding of plants and their healing properties. By respecting traditional knowledge while seeking scientific validation, herbalists can offer safe and effective treatments.

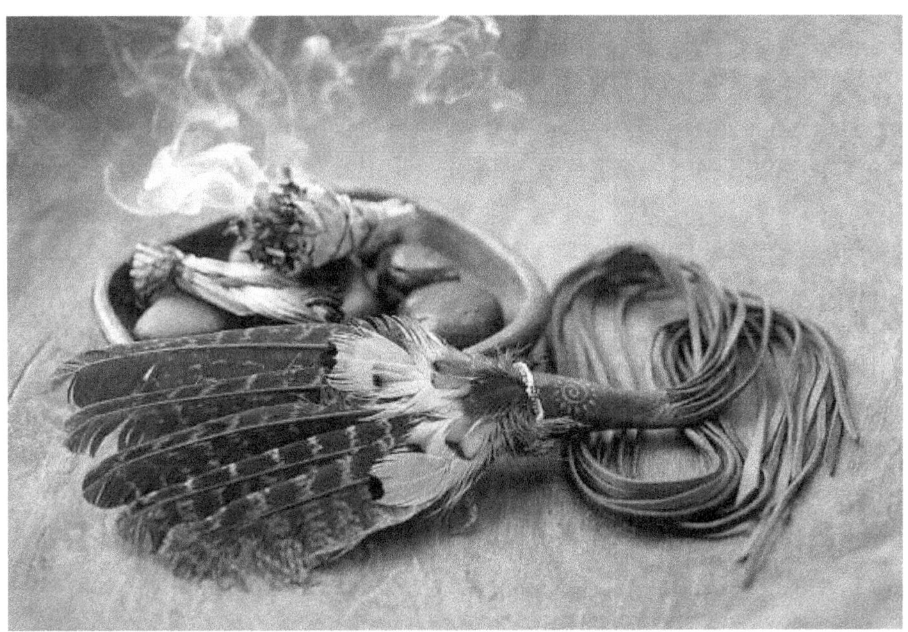

6. **Safety and Precautions:**

Herbal medicine recognizes that although herbs are natural substances, they can have potent effects on the body. Therefore, herbalists emphasize the importance of using herbs responsibly. This includes understanding proper dosages, potential interactions with medications or existing health conditions, and any contraindications. Herbalists prioritize the safety of their clients, taking precautions to minimize risks associated with herbal remedies. Conducting thorough consultations and considering an individual's unique circumstances helps ensure the safe and effective integration of herbal medicine into their healthcare routine.

7. **Sustainability and Conservation:**

Herbal medicine emphasizes the importance of sustainability and conservation efforts to ensure the availability of medicinal plants for future generations. With increasing global demand, responsible harvesting practices and the cultivation of endangered plants are paramount. Herbalists support ethical sources of herbal products and advocate for sustainable cultivation,
wildcrafting regulations, and initiatives promoting plant conservation. By embracing local plant remedies and fostering an appreciation for the natural abundance that surrounds us, herbalists contribute to the preservation of plant diversity and ecosystems.

8. **Collaboration with Conventional Medicine:**

Herbal medicine can complement conventional medical approaches by providing additional support and alternative options. Herbalists understand the benefits of working collaboratively with healthcare professionals, sharing knowledge, and integrating herbal remedies into conventional treatment plans when appropriate. By fostering an integrative approach, practitioners can combine the strengths of both herbal medicine and conventional medicine, maximizing patient outcomes and overall well-being.

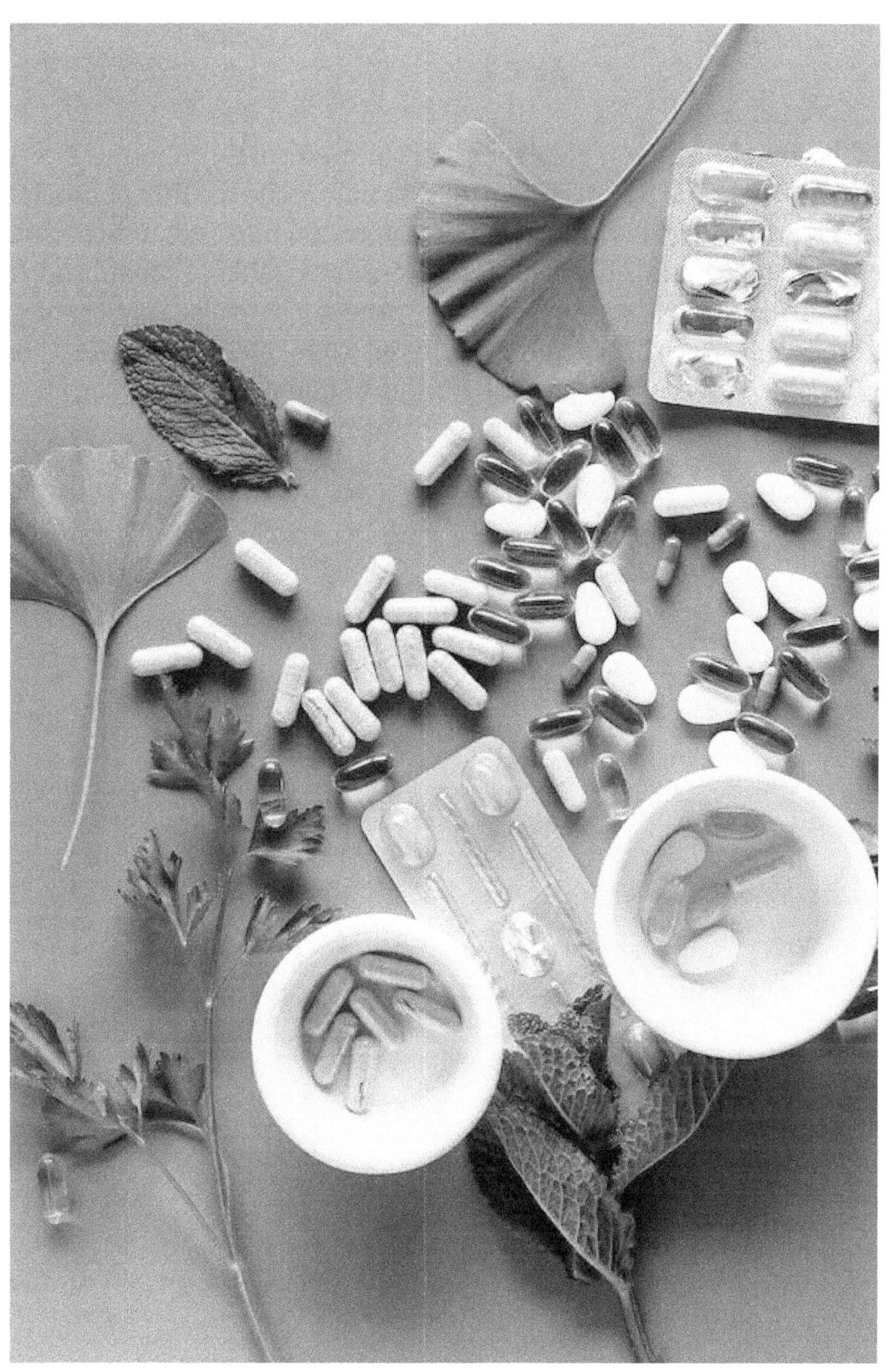

By embracing the principles of herbal medicine, individuals can embark on a journey of self-care and explore the healing potential of nature. It is important to remember that while herbal medicine can offer numerous benefits, it is always advisable to consult with a qualified herbalist or healthcare provider before incorporating herbs into a healthcare routine. This ensures the safe and effective integration of herbal medicine for individual needs, allowing for a holistic approach to health and well-being.

CHAPTER 4
Creating a Herbal Medicine Cabinet

When it comes to using herbal remedies, having a well-stocked herbal medicine cabinet is essential. Not only does it provide you with easy access to various herbs and remedies, but it also ensures that you are prepared for common ailments and health concerns that may arise. In this chapter, we will explore the key elements of creating a herbal medicine cabinet that is both comprehensive and effective.

1. Choosing the Right Herbs:

To create an effective herbal medicine cabinet, it's important to choose the right herbs that address your specific health needs. Here are some additional herbs that you can consider for various health issues:

Digestive   **Health:**

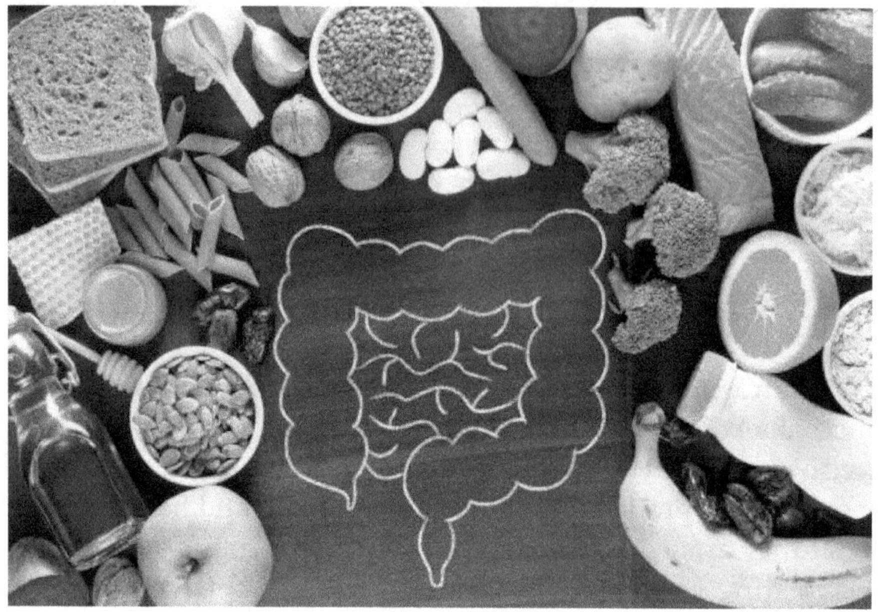

- ***Peppermint:*** In addition to its ability to soothe digestive discomforts, peppermint also has antispasmodic properties that help relieve intestinal cramps. It can be consumed as a tea, capsule, or added to culinary preparations.

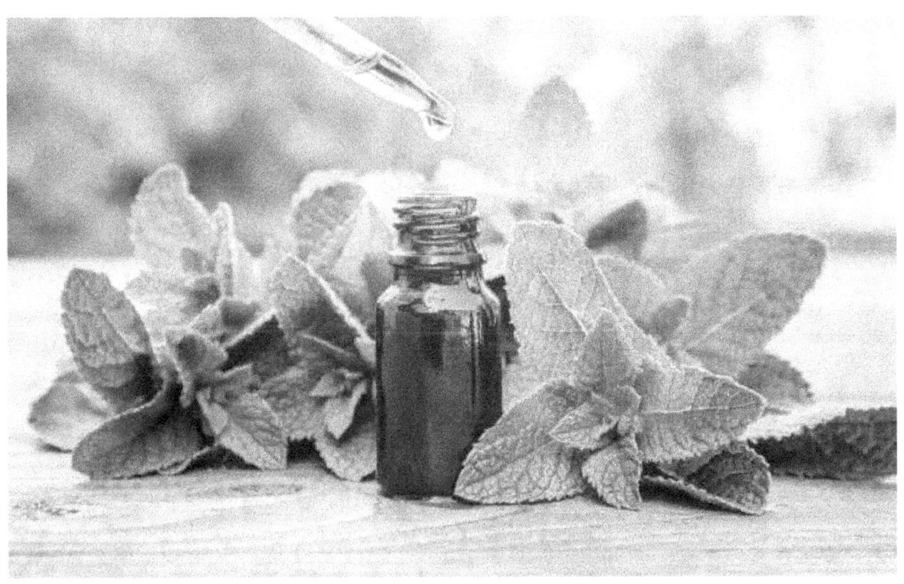

- ***Fennel:*** Known for its carminative and antispasmodic properties, fennel is excellent for relieving digestive issues like bloating, gas, and colic. Fennel seeds can be chewed or brewed into a tea after meals.

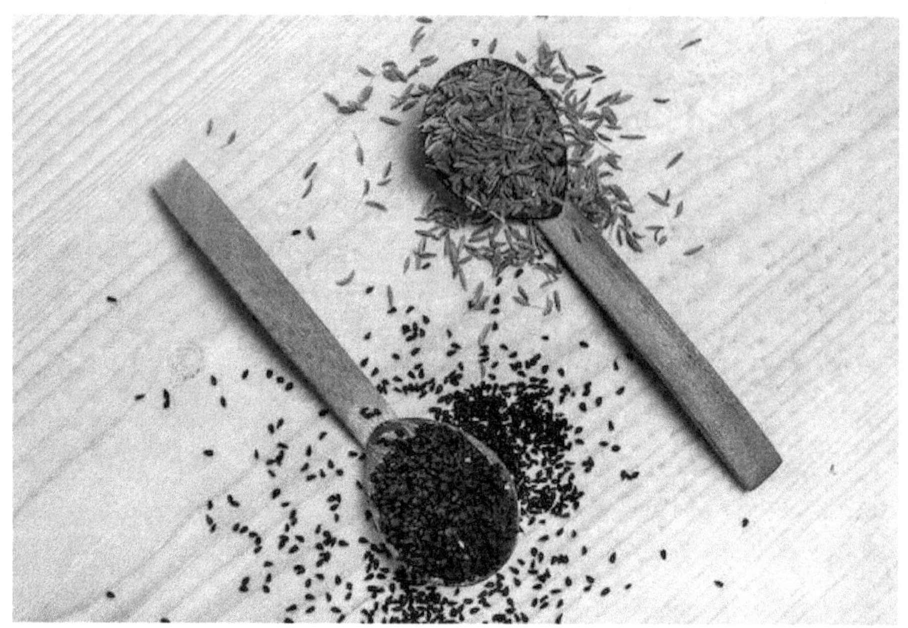

Respiratory Health:

- *Licorice Root:* Revered for its soothing and expectorant properties, licorice root is beneficial for respiratory conditions such as coughs, bronchitis, and sore throats. It can be consumed as a tea or in capsule form.

-

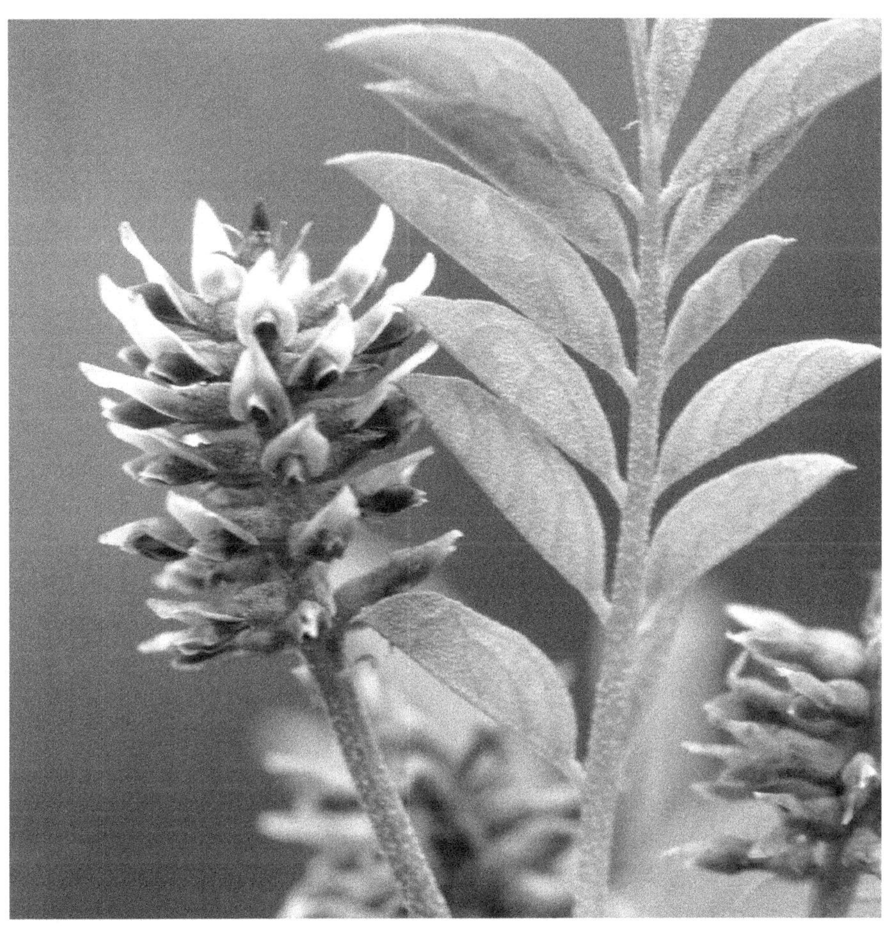

- *Mullein:* Mullein leaves have demulcent and expectorant properties, making them valuable for respiratory conditions like coughs, bronchitis, and asthma. Mullein tea or herbal infusions can be used to alleviate symptoms.

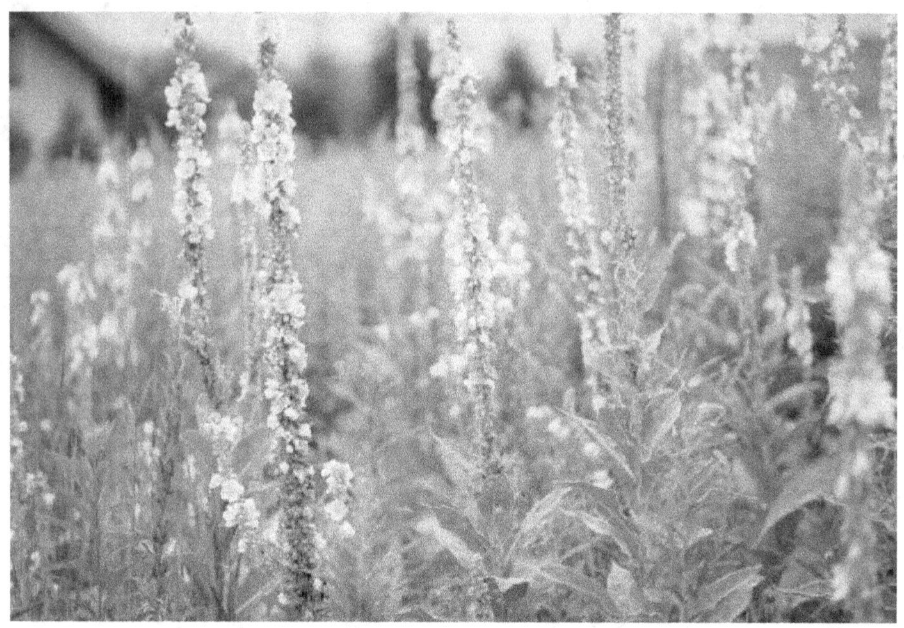

Immune Support:

- *Astragalus*: Often used in traditional Chinese medicine, astragalus has immune-modulating properties, making it a valuable herb for strengthening the immune system. Astragalus root can be brewed into tea or incorporated into culinary dishes.

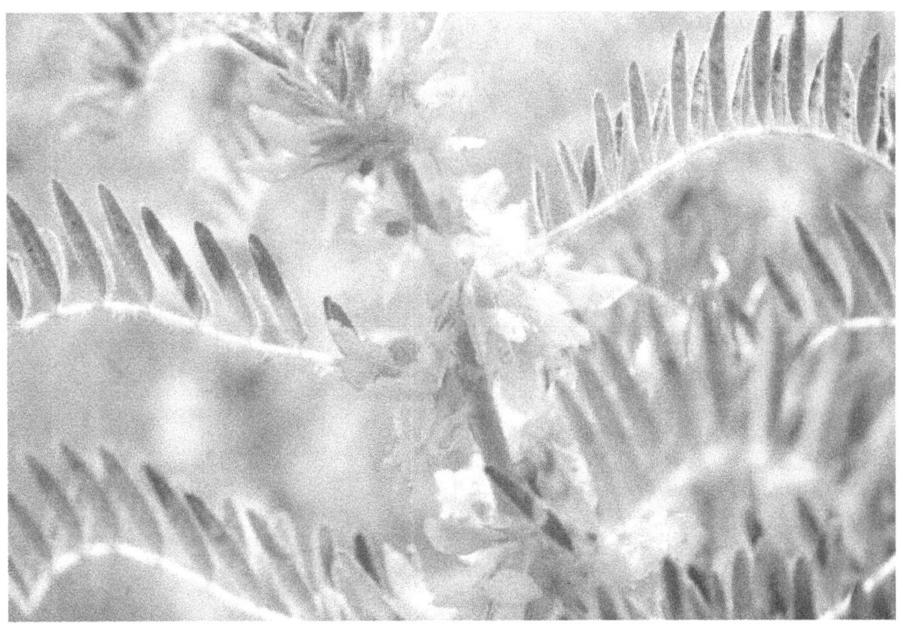

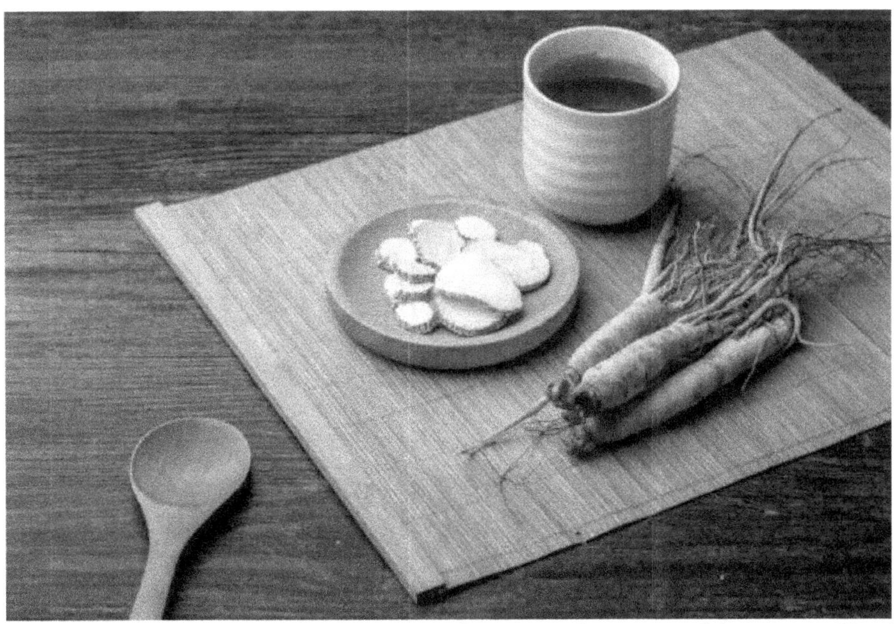

- ***Reishi Mushroom:*** Known as the "mushroom of immortality,"

reishi mushroom is believed to enhance immune function and reduce inflammation. Reishi mushrooms can be consumed as tea, powdered extract, or in capsules.

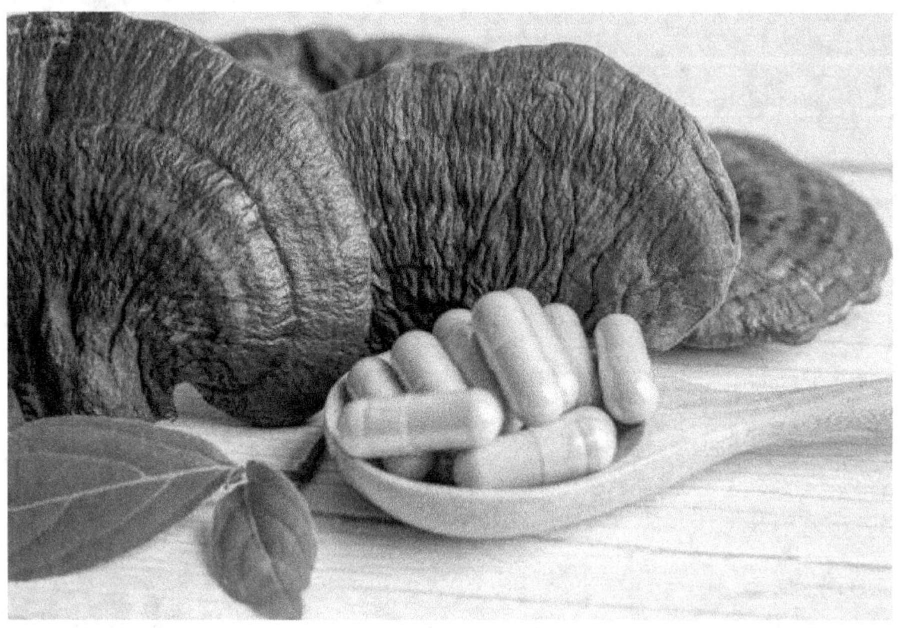

Stress Relief:

- *Lemon Balm:* Lemon balm is a calming herb that helps reduce anxiety, promote relaxation, and improve sleep quality.
It can be consumed as tea or tincture.

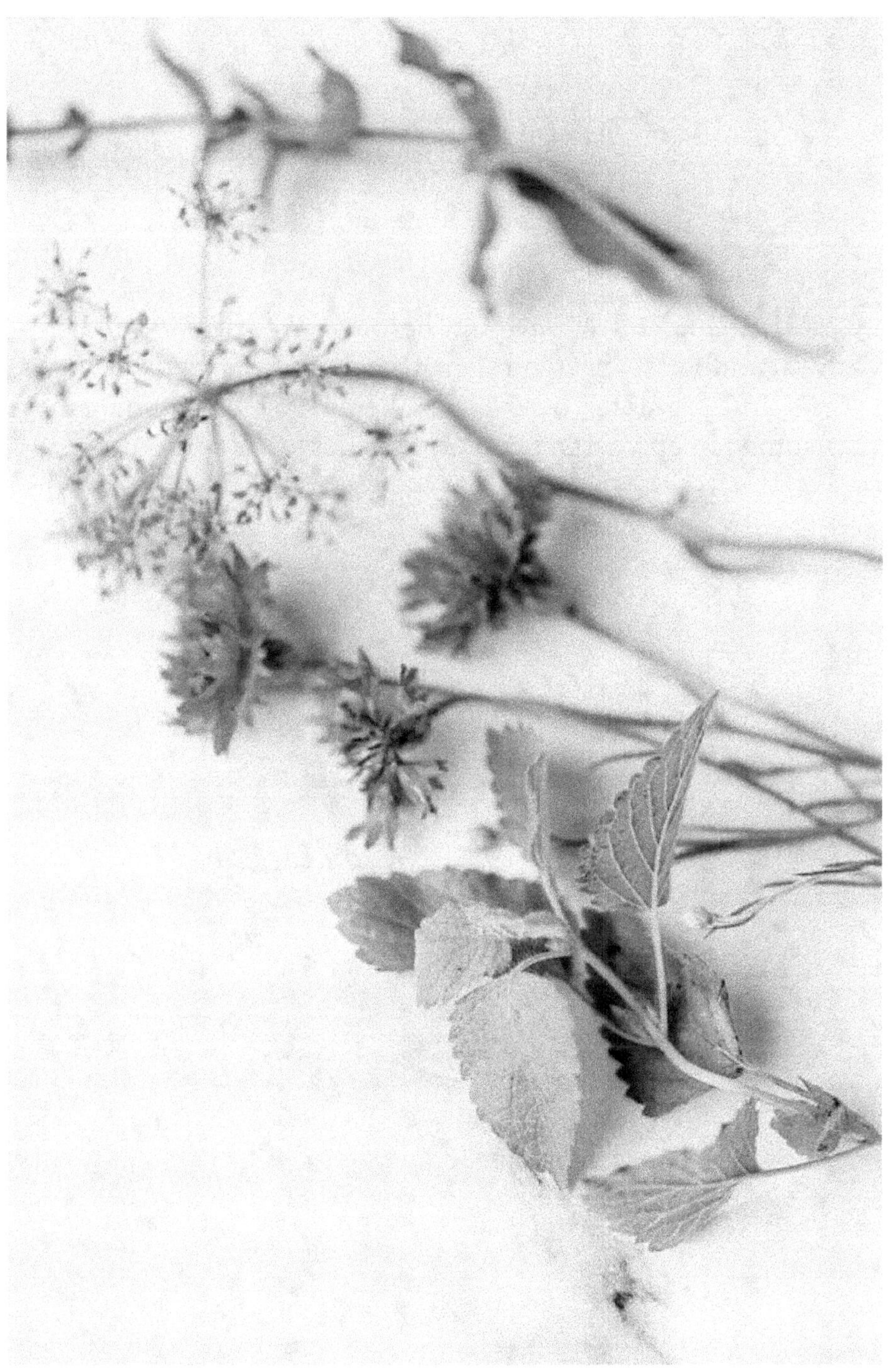

-

- ***Ashwagandha:*** A revered herb in Ayurvedic medicine, ashwagandha is an adaptogen that helps the body adapt to stress and promotes overall well-being. Ashwagandha can be consumed in powdered form, in capsules, or as a tincture.

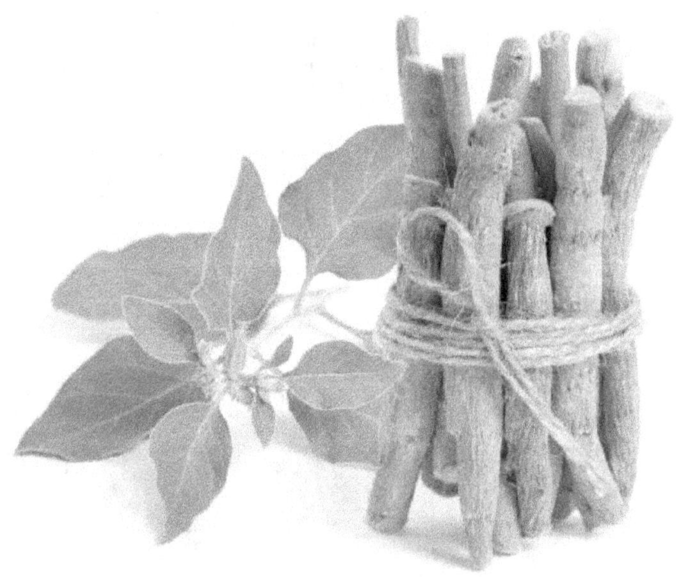

Skin Care:

- *Comfrey:* Comfrey is highly regarded for its ability to promote tissue repair and reduce inflammation, making it beneficial for skin conditions, cuts, and bruises. Comfrey can be used as a topical ointment or poultice.

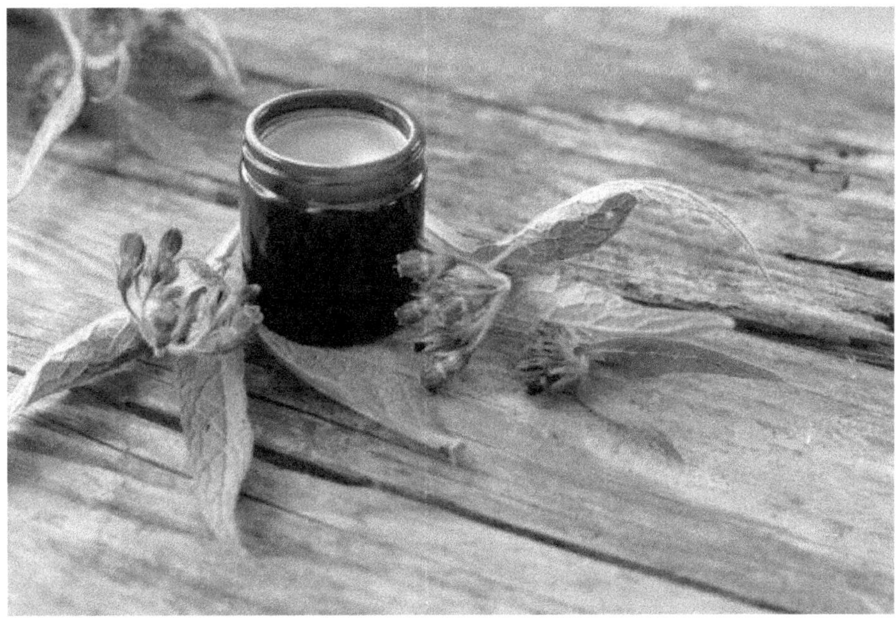

- ***Tea Tree Oil:*** With powerful antimicrobial and antiseptic properties, tea tree oil is excellent for treating various skin conditions like acne, fungal infections, and minor wounds. It can be applied topically in a diluted form.

2. **Storage and Organization:**

To maintain the potency and freshness of your herbs, proper storage and organization are crucial:

- - Choose storage containers that are airtight, light protected, and made of dark-tinted glass or high-quality plastic to prevent moisture, light, and air from deteriorating the herbs.
- - Label each container clearly with the herb's name, date of purchase, and any relevant details, such as the part of the herb used (leaves, flowers, roots, etc.), recommended dosage, and potential contraindications.
- -Store your herbal medicine cabinet in a cool, dry place away from direct sunlight and humidity. Consider investing in a spice rack or cabinet specifically designed for storing herbs.

3. Essential Tools and Supplies:

In addition to herbs, there are various essential tools and supplies to consider having in your herbal medicine cabinet:

1. - Mortar and Pestle: These traditional grinding tools are excellent for crushing and grinding herbs to extract their medicinal properties.
2. - Infusion Jars and Tea Strainers: Infusion jars are ideal for brewing herbal teas or creating single-herb infusions. Tea strainers or muslin cloth are essential for straining herbal preparations.
3. - Tincture Bottles: Tincture bottles are necessary for storing herbal extracts and tinctures for long-term use. Dark-tinted glass dropper bottles are typically used for this purpose.
4. - Carrier Oils: Carrier oils such as coconut oil, olive oil, or jojoba oil are crucial for making herbal salves, balms, and infused oils.
5. - Digital Scale: A digital scale ensures accurate measurement

of herb quantities, particularly when following herbal formulas or precise dosages.

6. - Reference Materials: It's invaluable to have reference materials such as herbal remedy books, plant identification guides, and reputable online resources to enhance your herbal knowledge and expand your range of remedies. **Safety Precautions:**

When using herbal remedies, it's important to take necessary safety precautions:

7. - Educate yourself about potential herb-drug interactions and contraindications. If you are currently taking medications or have underlying health conditions, consult a healthcare professional or herbalist before using herbal remedies.
8. - Use herbs within recommended dosages and durations specified by reliable sources or herbal practitioners.
9. -Keep your herbal medicine cabinet out of reach of children and pets.
10. - Keep a record of the herbs used, including the date of purchase, usage instructions, and any adverse reactions or side effects experienced. This record will help you track the effectiveness of remedies and inform healthcare professionals in case of emergencies (Abdulidha, et al. 2020).

By creating a well-stocked, organized, and carefully curated herbal medicine cabinet, you are empowering yourself to take control of your health and well-being. Regularly assess and replenish your supplies to ensure optimal potency and freshness. With the diverse range of herbs and essential tools at your disposal, you'll be well-prepared to address common ailments and promote overall wellness using the power of nature's remedies.

CHAPTER 5
Understanding Plant Identification and Harvesting

Plants have been used for medicinal purposes for thousands of years, and having a good understanding of plant identification and harvesting is crucial for safely and ethically utilizing herbs in herbal medicine. In this chapter, we will explore the various aspects of plant identification and harvesting to ensure that we are collecting the right plants at the right time and in the right way.

1. Importance of Proper Plant Identification:

- - Plant identification is essential to avoid misidentification, where the wrong plant is collected, potentially leading to harmful consequences.
- - Learn to identify plants through their unique characteristics such as leaves, stems, flowers, and overall growth habits.
- - Utilize reliable plant identification guides, and field manuals, or consult with local experts to improve accuracy.
- - Develop a systematic approach to verify identification by cross-referencing multiple sources and confirming through direct observation.

2. Researching Plant Habitat and Seasonality:

- - Each plant species has specific habitat preferences and seasonal growth patterns.

• - Familiarize yourself with the preferred habitats and growing conditions of the plants you are interested in.
• - Understand the optimal time to harvest each plant, as this can greatly affect its medicinal properties.
• - Consider factors such as altitude, soil type, moisture levels, and exposure to sunlight when identifying suitable plant habitats.
• - Keep records of plant sightings and note any variations in habitat or growth patterns to deepen your understanding of plant behavior.

3. Ethical and Sustainable Harvesting Practices:

• - Harvesting ethically and sustainably protects plant populations and ensures their continued growth.
• - Only collect plants that are abundant and not threatened or endangered.
• - Observe proper foraging etiquette, such as asking for permission to harvest on private property or obtaining necessary permits in protected areas.
• - Stay informed about local regulations and guidelines regarding wild harvesting to ensure compliance with legal and conservation measures.
• - Harvest in moderation, leaving enough plants for natural propagation and ecological balance.
• - Adopt a "take only what you need" mentality to minimize your impact on the ecosystem.
• - Consider participating in local conservation efforts supporting sustainable cultivation practices to contribute positively to plant conservation.

4. Tools and Techniques for Harvesting:

• - Invest in good quality tools such as pruners, shears, or scissors for harvesting plant material.

- - Ensure your tools are sharp to make clean cuts with minimal damage to the plant.
- - Practice proper hygiene by cleaning tools before and after use to prevent the spread of pests or diseases.
- - Use appropriate tools based on the plant's growth habit– for example, pruners for woody plants and scissors for delicate or herbaceous plants.
- - Consider using a harvesting knife or scissors with a serrated edge to facilitate precise cutting and minimize damage.
- - Harvest above the growth point or node to allow the plant to regenerate more easily.

- - Support the health of the plant by removing any dead or diseased parts during the harvesting process.

5. Preserving Harvested Plants:

- - After harvesting, it is important to preserve the plants to maintain their potency and longevity.
- - Proper drying techniques are essential to prevent the growth of mold or bacteria and preserve the medicinal properties of the plants.
- - Air drying is a common method, but you can also use a dehydrator or dry herbs in the oven on low heat.
- - Spread harvested plant material in a single layer on drying racks or screens to ensure adequate airflow.
- - Monitor the drying process by regularly checking the plants for dryness and removing any moldy or damaged material.
- - Store the dried plants in airtight containers made of glass, ceramic, or metal to protect them from light, moisture, and pests.
- - Consider labeling the containers with the plant name, date of harvest, and any important details or observations.
- - Explore other preservation methods like making tinctures, oils, syrups, or herbal vinegar to expand the range of applications and storage options.

6. Documenting and Cataloging:

- - Keeping a detailed record of the plants you harvest enhances your knowledge and allows for future reference and research.
- - Note the location, date, and specific part of the plant collected, as well as any important observations or experiences during the harvesting process.
- - Consider creating a digital or physical catalog with photographs, sketches, or descriptions of the plants you encounter.
- - Include information on the plant's growth habit, preferred habitat, uses, and any related folklore or traditional knowledge.
- - Share your catalog or findings with other herbalists or enthusiasts to contribute to collective knowledge about medicinal plants.
- - Continuously revisit and update your catalog as you learn and discover more about plant identification and harvesting techniques.

By thoroughly understanding plant identification and harvesting techniques, you can confidently collect and utilize medicinal plants for your herbal remedies. Approach this process with respect for nature and the plants themselves, ensuring sustainability and long-term availability of these valuable resources. Remember that continuous learning, observation, and collaboration with experienced herbalists can further enhance your skills in plant identification and harvesting. Taking the time to delve deeper into these topics will allow you to connect more profoundly with the natural world and its therapeutic gifts.

CHAPTER 6
Herbal Preparation Methods

In this chapter, we will explore the various methods of preparing herbal remedies to harness their healing properties. Understanding the different preparation techniques is crucial for extracting the beneficial compounds from the plants effectively. Let's delve into some commonly used methods:

1. Infusions and Decoctions:

Infusions and Decoctions are simple and widely used methods of extracting the medicinal properties of herbs. Infusions involve steeping herbs in hot water, whereas Decoctions involve simmering herbs in water for a prolonged period. These methods are suitable for extracting both water-soluble and heat-stable compounds, allowing for a broader range of medicinal benefits.

To make an infusion, typically used for delicate plant parts like leaves and flowers, boil water and pour it over the herbs in a covered container. Let it steep for the recommended time, usually 5-10 minutes, strain, and enjoy as a tea or use for external applications. Infusions can also be cold brewed by soaking herbs in cold water overnight, providing a milder flavor.

Decoctions, on the other hand, are excellent for tougher plant materials like roots, bark, and seeds. Simmer the herbs in water for 15-30 minutes, ensuring the liquid reduces to extract the desired compounds. Strain the decoction and use it according to the specific remedies. Decoctions can be refrigerated and reheated or used as a base for herbal soups, syrups, and syrups.

2. Tinctures:

Tinctures are concentrated herbal extracts that use alcohol as a solvent. This method is particularly useful for preserving the medicinal properties of the herbs for an extended period. Alcohol extracts a wide range of compounds, including essential oils, alkaloids, glycosides, and flavonoids.

To create a tincture, select a high-quality botanical material and finely grind or chop it. Place the herb in a glass jar and cover it completely with a high-proof alcohol, such as vodka or brandy. The ideal alcohol concentration is around 40-60%, as it effectively extracts a broad range of compounds. Seal the jar tightly and leave it to macerate for several weeks, shaking it daily. The maceration period allows the alcohol to dissolve the active constituents from the plant material.

After the maceration period, strain the liquid through the cheese-

cloth or a fine sieve, pressing the herb to extract as much liquid as possible. The resulting liquid is tincture, which can be stored in dark glass bottles with dropper caps for easy and precise dosage. Tinctures have a longer shelf life compared to other herbal preparations and can be used internally or externally by diluting them in water or other beverages.

3. Herbal Oils:

Herbal oils are created by infusing plant material in a carrier oil, such as olive oil or coconut oil. This method is ideal for extracting essential oils, as well as other beneficial compounds present in herbs. The resulting infused oils can be used for massage, topical application, or as a base for salves and lotions.

To make herbal oil, finely chop or grind the dried herbs and mix them with the carrier oil. The ratio of herbs to oil varies depending on the desired potency, but a common guideline is a 1:5 or 1:10 ratio. Ensure that the herbs are fully submerged in the oil to prevent spoilage. Place the mixture in a glass jar and store it in a warm area for several weeks, gently shaking it every day to promote infusion.

After the allotted time, strain the oil using cheesecloth or a fine sieve, squeezing out as much oil as possible. The resulting infused oil can be stored in dark glass bottles and used topically by gently massaging it into the skin. Herbal oils can also be used as carriers for essential oils or as a base for ointments, creams, and salves.

4. Poultices and Compresses:

Poultices and compresses involve directly applying fresh or dried herbs to the affected area of the body. Poultices are made by crushing or grinding fresh herbs and applying them directly to the skin, while compresses involve soaking a cloth in an herbal infusion or Decoctions and applying it as a warm or cold pack.

To create a poultice, select fresh herbs known for their healing properties, such as comfrey leaves or plantain. Finely chop or crush the herbs and apply them directly to the affected area. Cover with a cloth or bandage to hold the poultice in place and leave it on for the recommended time, usually 1530 minutes. Poultices are beneficial for treating minor wounds, relieving insect bites, reducing inflammation, and soothing skin irritations.

Compresses, on the other hand, work by applying the herbal infusion or Decoctions directly to the affected area using a cloth soaked in the liquid. For a warm compress, soak a cloth in a hot herbal infusion, gently wring out excess liquid, and apply it to the affected area. This method is often used to relieve muscle aches, joint pain, and swelling. For a cold compress, follow the same steps using a cold infusion or refrigerate the compress before application to reduce inflammation, ease headaches, or soothe sunburns.

5. Syrups and Elixirs:

Syrups and elixirs are sweet liquid preparations that combine herbs with honey, sugar, or another sweetener. These preparations are often used to make herbal remedies more palatable, especially for children. Syrups are made by simmering an herbal infusion or Decoctions with sweeteners until they reach a thick and syrupy consistency, usually using a 1:1 ratio of liquid to sweetener.

To make a syrup, start by preparing an herbal infusion or Decoctions using the desired herbs. Simmer the liquid until it reduces by half and strain out any solids. Add an equal amount of sweetener, such as honey or maple syrup, to the strained liquid while it's still warm, stirring until the sweetener dissolves completely. Once cooled, pour the syrup into a sterilized glass jar, and store it in the refrigerator. Syrups are commonly used to alleviate coughs and sore throats and as immune system boosters.

Elixirs, on the other hand, involve combining herbal tinctures with sweeteners for a concentrated and easily dosed remedy. Start by selecting the desired herbal tinctures and determine the appropriate ratios for each. Combine the tinctures in a glass jar and add the sweetener of choice, such as glycerin or honey, until the desired taste is achieved. Close the jar securely and gently shake it to mix the ingredients thoroughly. Elixirs can be taken orally by themselves or added to beverages and are commonly used for various health-promoting purposes.

6. Capsules and Tablets:

For those who prefer a more convenient and portable form of herbal remedies, capsules and tablets are popular options. These preparations involve encapsulating powdered herbs or compressing them into tablet form. This method allows for precise dosing and easy storage, making it suitable for long-term use or travel.

To create capsules, start by grinding dried herbs into a fine powder using a mortar and pestle or a coffee grinder dedicated to herbal preparations. Once the herbs are finely powdered, use a capsule-filling machine or manual capsule-filling device to fill empty gelatin or vegetarian capsules with the powdered herb. The capsules can be purchased from herbal suppliers or health stores. Fill the capsules with the desired amount of powdered herb, ensuring they are tightly packed, and then secure the capsules by snapping the two halves together. Store the filled capsules in a dark glass jar or airtight container.

Tablets, on the other hand, require a tablet press machine to compress the powdered herbs into tablet form. This method involves mixing the powdered herb with a binder, such as gum Arabic or cellulose, to ensure the tablets hold their shape. The mixture is then compressed into tablet form using the tablet press machine, creating uniform tablets that can be easily swallowed. Tablets are often made in larger batches, making them a convenient option for long-term use or to share with others.

Both capsules and tablets offer a convenient and discreet way to take herbal remedies. They can be easily stored, carried, and taken with water or other beverages. However, it's important to note that capsules and tablets may take longer to assimilate in the body compared to other forms of herbal preparations, as the body needs to break them down before absorption can occur.

Each method of herbal preparation has its own unique advantages and is suitable for different situations or personal preferences. It's important to choose the appropriate preparation method based on the specific herb and its desired medicinal benefits. Experimenting with different techniques can help you discover the most effective and enjoyable way to incorporate herbal remedies into your daily routine.

CHAPTER 7

Healing Herbs for Common Ailments

Herbal medicine has been used for centuries to treat a wide range of common ailments. From the flu to headaches and digestive issues, there are many herbs known for their healing properties. In this chapter, we will explore some of these herbs in depth and discuss how they can be used to alleviate various health conditions.

1. Echinacea (Echinacea purpurea):

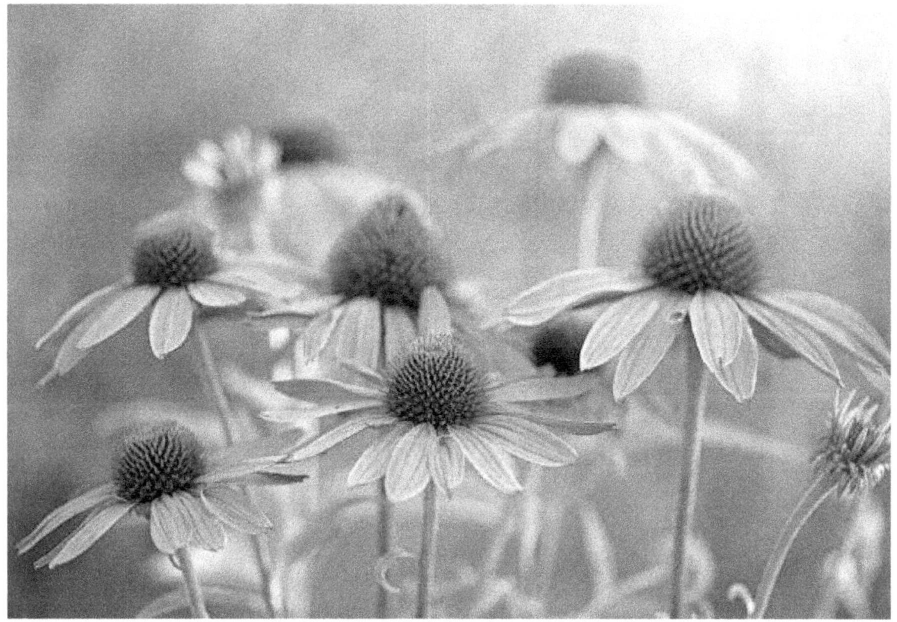

Echinacea is a fascinating herb known for its immune-boosting properties. It stimulates the production of white blood cells and activates natural killer cells, enhancing the body's ability to fight off infections. Echinacea can be particularly effective in preventing and treating respiratory tract infections, such as the common cold and flu. It also has antiviral and antibacterial properties that further support its immune-stimulating effects.

Echinacea is available in various forms, including teas, tinctures, capsules, and extracts. For acute illnesses, it is recommended to take Echinacea at the first sign of symptoms and continue for a few days or until symptoms subside. However, it's important to note that prolonged use of Echinacea may decrease its effectiveness, so it is best to use it intermittently. People with autoimmune disorders or allergies to ragweed should consult with their healthcare provider before using Echinacea.

2. Ginger (Zingiber officinale):

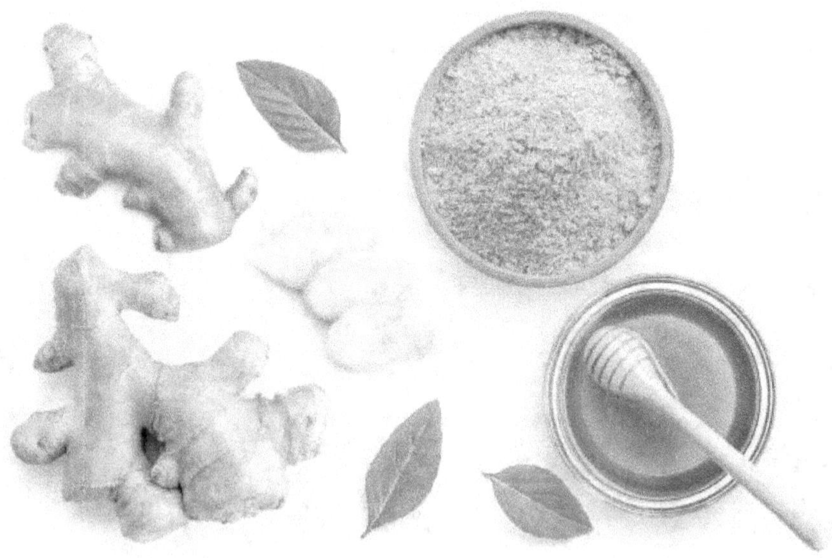

Ginger is a versatile and widely used herb, well-known for its digestive benefits and anti-inflammatory properties. It contains compounds called gingerols and shogaols that help calm the stomach, relieve nausea, and reduce inflammation in the gastrointestinal tract. Ginger is commonly used to treat digestive discomfort, including indigestion, bloating, and nausea.

Moreover, ginger has shown promise in reducing symptoms of motion sickness, morning sickness during pregnancy, and chemotherapy-induced nausea. It can also be beneficial in reducing menstrual pain and migraines due to its ability to block prostaglandin synthesis and alleviate inflammation.

Ginger can be consumed in various forms, including fresh ginger root, ginger tea, capsules, or as an ingredient in meals. However, individuals taking blood-thinning medications or those with gallstones should exercise caution and consult with a healthcare provider before using ginger regularly.

3.   **Chamomile (Matricaria chamomilla):**

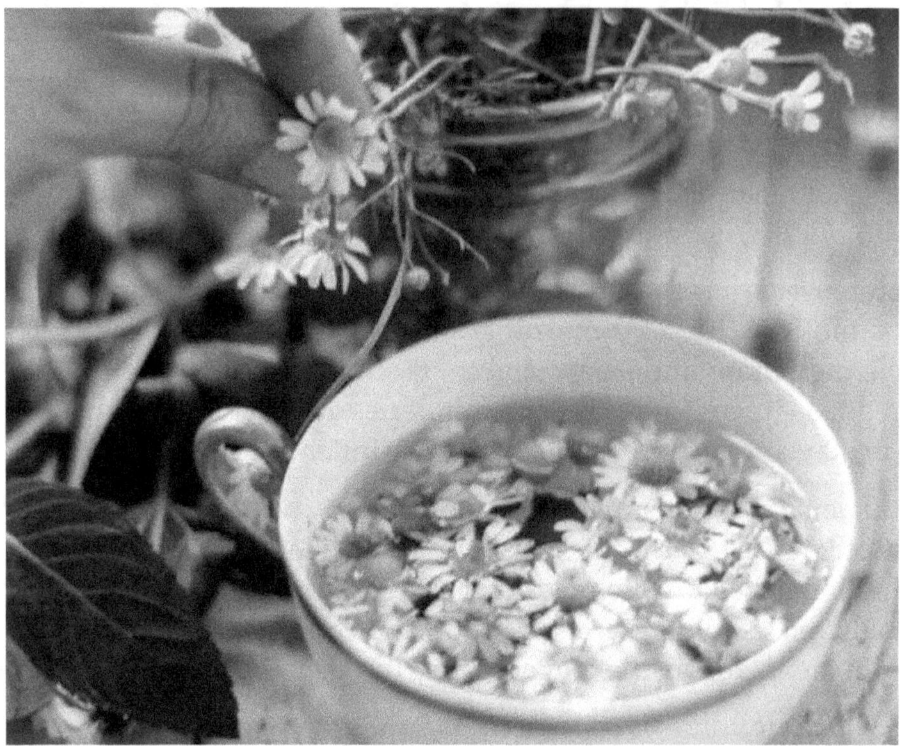

Chamomile is a gentle and soothing herb that has been used for centuries to promote relaxation and improve sleep quality. It contains compounds such as bisabolol and chamazulene, which possess anti-inflammatory properties, making it beneficial for a variety of conditions.

Chamomile tea is most consumed to induce sleep and reduce anxiety. It has a mild sedative effect that can calm the nervous system, making it useful for those with insomnia or high levels of stress. Apart from its sleep-enhancing properties, chamomile tea has also been found to relieve symptoms of irritable bowel syndrome (IBS). Its antispasmodic and anti-inflammatory effects can help soothe the gastrointestinal tract and reduce cramping and bloating.

Topically, chamomile can be used as a rinse or poultice to treat skin irritations, such as eczema and minor wounds, due to its anti-inflammatory and antimicrobial properties. However, individuals with allergies to ragweed or related plants should avoid chamomile.

4. Peppermint (Mentha piperita):

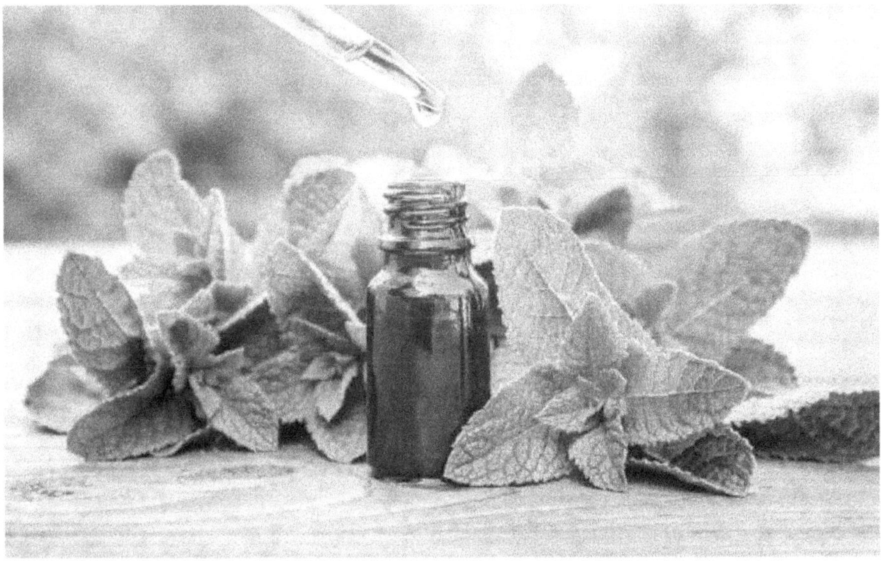

Peppermint is a refreshing herb that has long been used for its digestive and pain-relieving properties. It contains an active compound called menthol, which provides a cooling and calming effect on the body. Peppermint is commonly used to soothe upset stomachs, relieve headaches, and reduce muscle pain.

Peppermint tea or oil can be consumed to alleviate digestive discomfort, including indigestion, bloating, and gas. The volatile oils in peppermint can relax the muscles of the gastrointestinal tract, promoting healthy digestion and reducing symptoms of irritable bowel syndrome (IBS).

When used topically, peppermint essential oil can provide relief for tension headaches and muscle aches. However, it should be used with caution in infants and young children, as it may cause breathing difficulties, and individuals with gastroesophageal reflux disease (GERD) may experience increased acid reflux symptoms.

5. Turmeric (Curcuma longa):

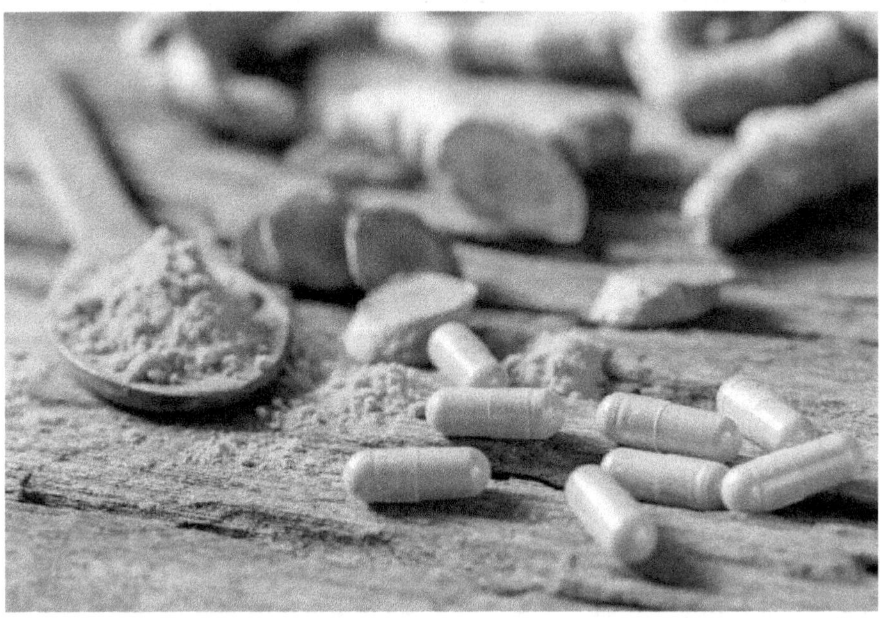

Turmeric is a vibrant yellow spice widely used in cooking and traditional medicine. Its main active compound, curcumin, possesses potent anti-inflammatory and antioxidant effects. Turmeric has been used for centuries to reduce pain and inflammation associated with various conditions, including arthritis and joint pain.

Curcumin's anti-inflammatory properties extend to other areas of the body as well, making it a potential aid in reducing the risk of chronic diseases like heart disease, diabetes, and cancer. It can modulate several signaling pathways involved in inflammation, oxidative stress, and cell growth.

Turmeric can be incorporated into meals by adding it to curries, soups, or smoothies. However, curcumin is not easily absorbed by the body, so it is often recommended to consume turmeric with black pepper or in combination with fats, such as coconut oil or olive oil, for optimal absorption.

6. Lavender (Lavandula angustifolia):

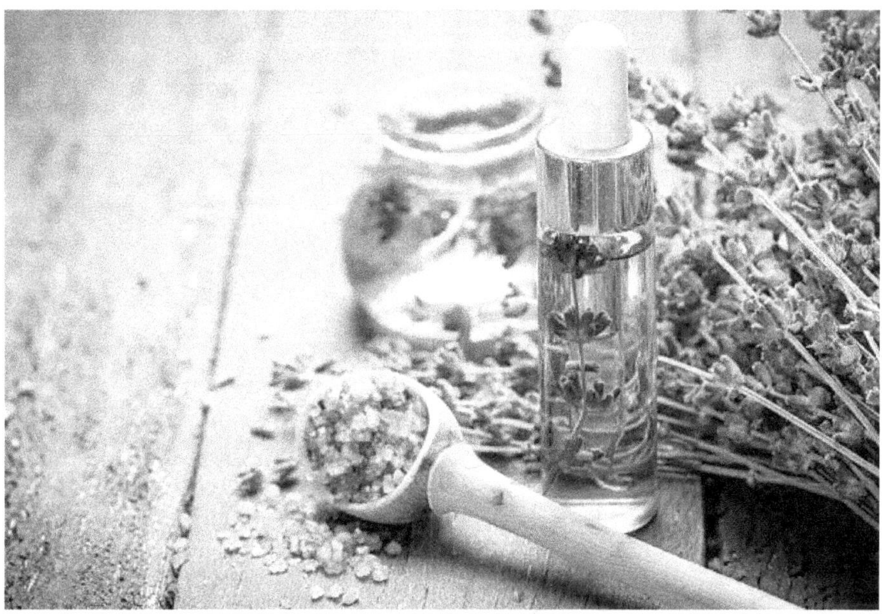

Lavender is a beautiful herb often associated with relaxation, tranquility, and sleep. Its calming effects make it popular in aromatherapy and as an additive in bath products. The scent of lavender has been shown to lower heart rate and blood pressure, promoting a sense of calmness, and reducing stress and anxiety.

In addition to its calming properties, lavender essential oil possesses antibacterial and anti-fungal properties, making it useful for minor cuts, burns, and skin irritations. It can also be soothing for conditions such as eczema and insect bites.

The lavender essential oil can be used in a diffuser, added to bathwater, or applied topically (diluted with a carrier oil) for relaxation and wound healing benefits. However, caution should be exercised, as some individuals may experience allergic reactions or skin irritation.

7. **Garlic (Allium sativum):**

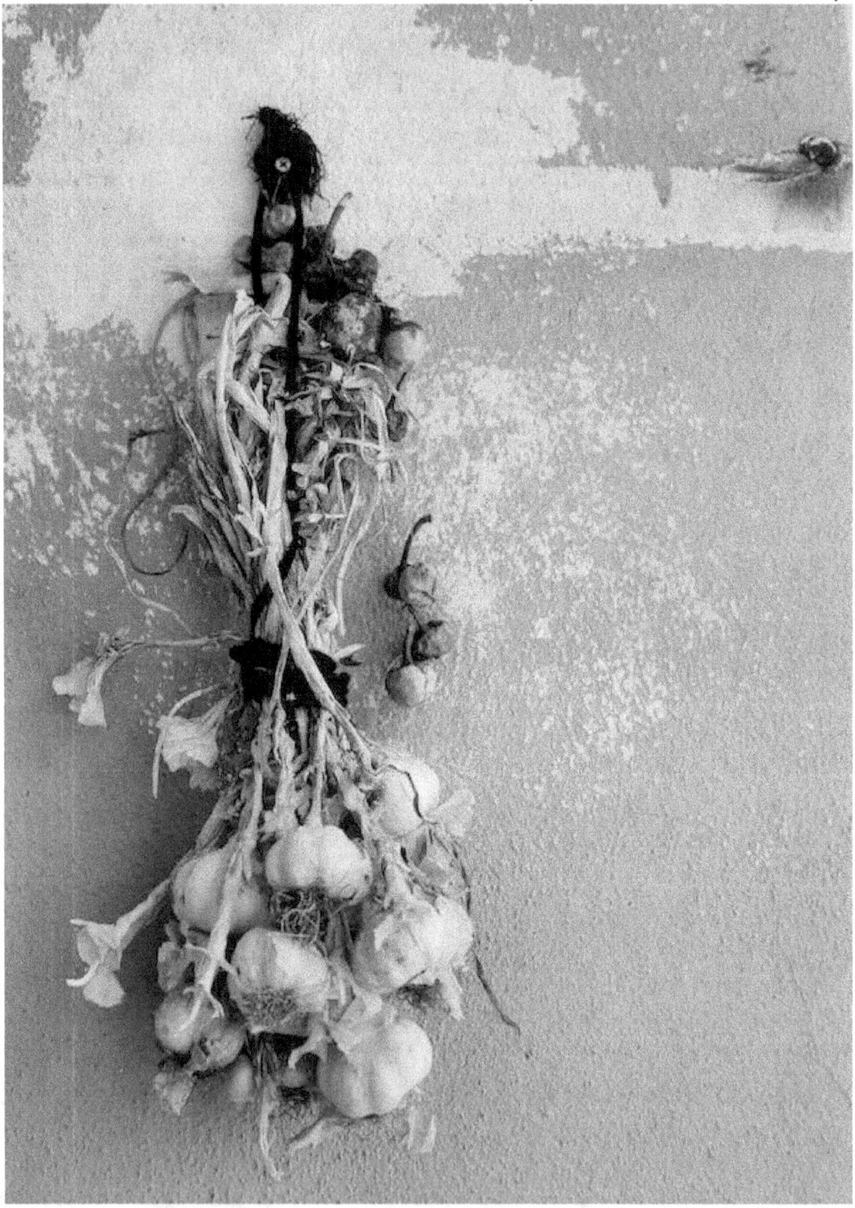

Garlic is a pungent herb that not only adds flavor to many dishes but also offers numerous health benefits. It has been used for centuries as a natural remedy due to its immune-boosting properties and ability to fight off infections. Garlic contains a compound called allicin, which exhibits antimicrobial and antifungal properties and may be effective against bacteria, viruses, and fungi.

Garlic is commonly used to support respiratory health and prevent the common cold and flu. It can also be beneficial for cardiovascular health by reducing blood pressure, lowering cholesterol levels, and improving blood circulation. Additionally, garlic has been shown to have anticancer properties and may help lower the risk of certain types of cancer.

To harness the benefits of garlic, it is best to consume it raw or crushed to activate the release of allicin. However, garlic may interact with certain medications, particularly blood-thinning medication, and should be used with caution in individuals with bleeding disorders or who are about to undergo surgery.

8. **Valerian (Valeriana officinalis):**

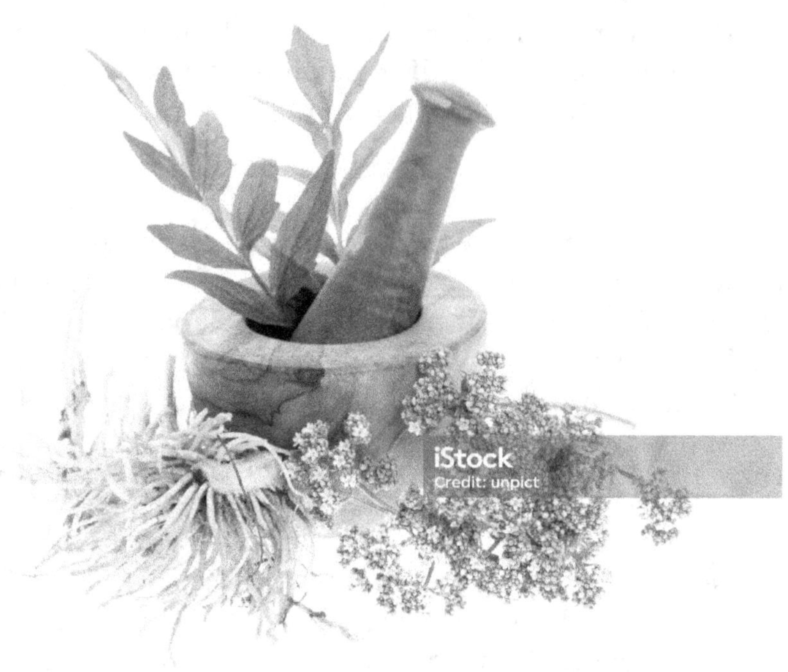

Valerian root is an herb commonly used to promote relaxation and treat insomnia. It has been used for centuries as a natural sleep aid due to its calming and sedative effects. Valerian interacts with the GABA receptors in the brain, which helps to reduce anxiety and promote a sense of calmness.

Valerian can be consumed as a tea or in supplement form. It is often recommended to take Valerian supplements about an hour before bedtime to help induce sleep. It may take a few weeks of regular use to experience the full benefits of Valerian, so it is important to be consistent with its use.

While Valerian is generally safe for short-term use, long-term use or high doses may result in side effects such as headaches, dizziness, or gastrointestinal upset. It is important to consult with a healthcare provider before using Valerian, especially if you are taking other medications or have an underlying medical condition.

9. St. John's Wort (Hypericum perforatum):

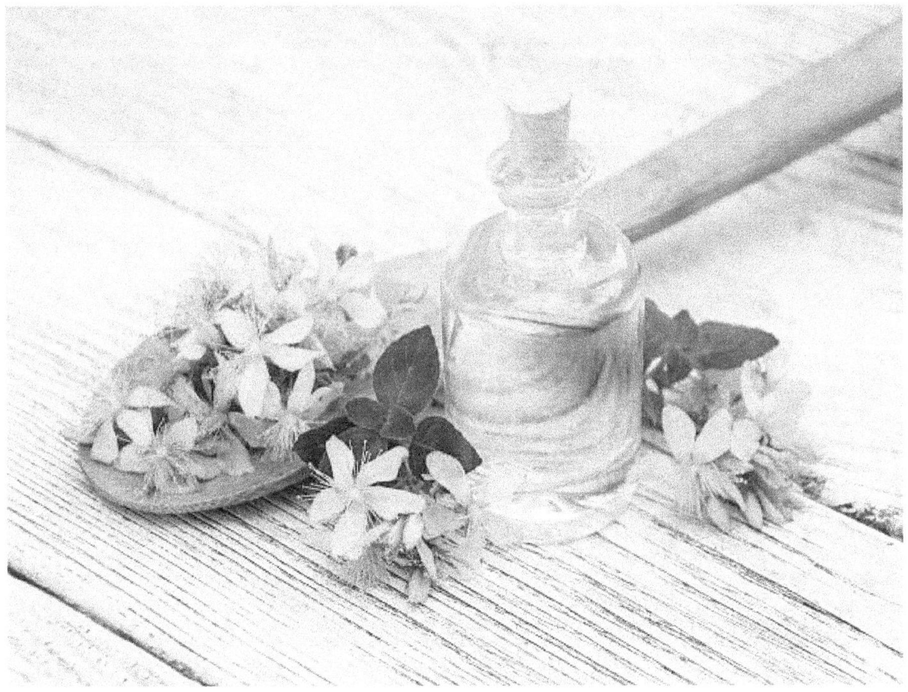

St. John's Wort is an herb that has been traditionally used to treat depression and promote emotional well-being. It contains various active compounds, including hypericin and hyperforin, which are believed to be responsible for its antidepressant effects.

St. John's Wort may help alleviate symptoms of mild to moderate depression, such as low mood, sadness, and anxiety. It works by increasing the levels of certain neurotransmitters, such as serotonin, in the brain. However, it is important to note that St. John's Wort can interact with certain medications, including antidepressants, birth control pills, and blood-thinning medications. It is essential to consult with a healthcare provider before using St. John's Wort to ensure it is safe for your specific situation.

10. Calendula (Calendula officinalis):

Calendula, also known as marigold, is a beautiful herb with vibrant orange flowers. It has been used for centuries for its medicinal properties, particularly for its ability to soothe and heal the skin.

Calendula has anti-inflammatory and antimicrobial properties, making it beneficial for various skin conditions, including cuts, scrapes, burns, and rashes. It can help reduce swelling, promote wound healing, and prevent infections. Calendula is applied topically as a cream, ointment, or infused oil to the affected area.

Additionally, calendula tea can be consumed to support digestive health and reduce inflammation in the gastrointestinal tract. It can help relieve symptoms of gastritis, gastric ulcers, and colitis.

Calendula tea can be enjoyed alone or combined with other medicinal herbs for enhanced benefits.

Herbal medicine offers a wide range of healing herbs that can be used to alleviate common ailments. From immune-boosting Echinacea to digestive-soothing ginger and sleep-promoting chamomile, these herbs provide natural alternatives for addressing various health conditions. However, it is important to note that herbs are not a substitute for medical advice or treatment. If you have any concerns or pre-existing health conditions, it is best to consult with a healthcare provider before using herbs for medicinal purposes.

CHAPTER 8
Herbal Remedies for Digestive Health

The digestive system plays a vital role in our overall well-being. When it is functioning properly, we can efficiently absorb nutrients and eliminate waste. However, digestive issues such as indigestion, bloating, and constipation can greatly affect our quality of life. Fortunately, nature offers a plethora of herbs that can support and promote digestive health. In this chapter, we will delve even deeper into the world of herbal remedies for digestive issues, exploring their mechanisms of action and additional benefits.

1. Peppermint (Mentha piperita):

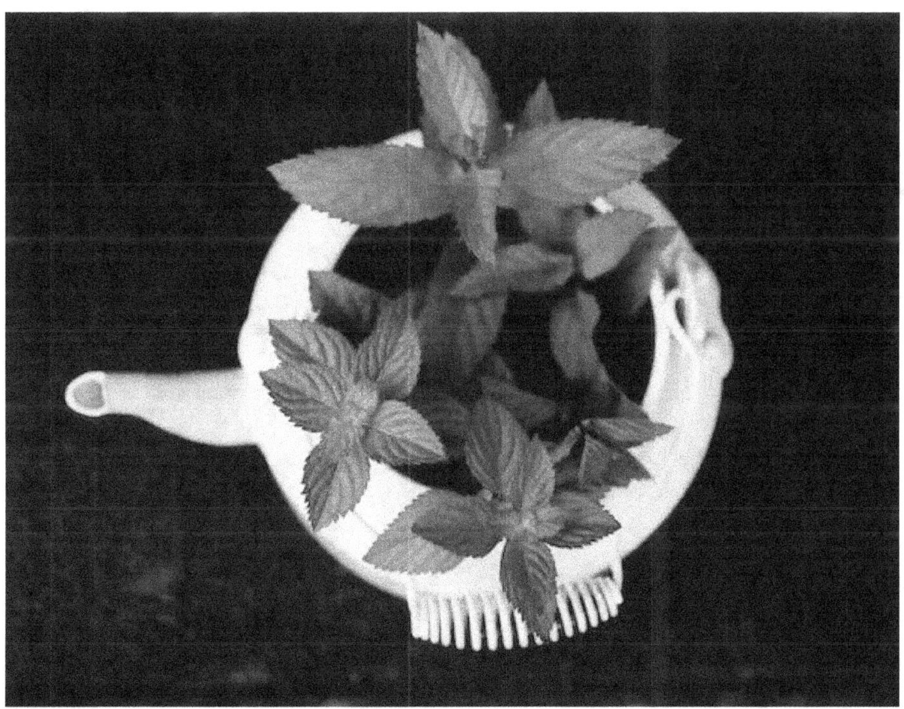

Peppermint is widely known for its soothing properties on the digestive system. It contains an active compound called menthol, which helps relax the muscles of the gastrointestinal tract, relieving symptoms of indigestion, bloating, and gas. Peppermint can also aid in reducing symptoms of irritable bowel syndrome (IBS) by reducing muscle spasms in the colon. Additionally, peppermint has analgesic properties, which can help ease abdominal pain. Clinical studies have shown its efficacy in improving symptoms of digestive disorders. You can enjoy the therapeutic benefits of peppermint by drinking peppermint tea, utilizing peppermint essential oil in aromatherapy, or taking it in capsule form.

2. Ginger (Zingiber officinale):

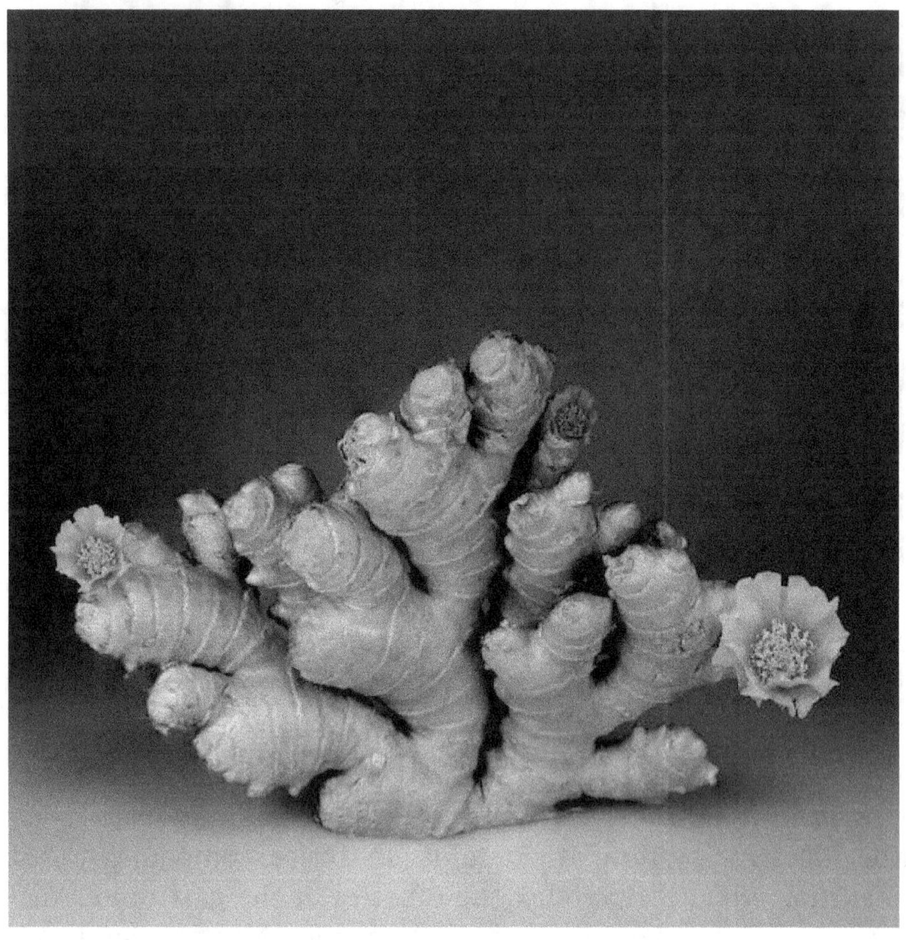

Ginger has been used medicinally for centuries to aid digestion. Its strong anti-inflammatory properties help reduce inflammation in the gastrointestinal tract, alleviating symptoms of nausea, bloating, and indigestion. Ginger also stimulates the production of digestive enzymes, aiding in the breakdown of food and promoting optimal absorption of nutrients. Moreover, ginger can help relieve motion sickness and reduce postoperative nausea and vomiting. Its analgesic properties make it useful in easing menstrual cramps and migraines. Recent studies have also suggested its potential in preventing certain types of cancer. To incorporate ginger into your routine, you can enjoy ginger tea, chew on fresh ginger, or take it in capsule form.

3. Fennel (Foeniculum vulgare):

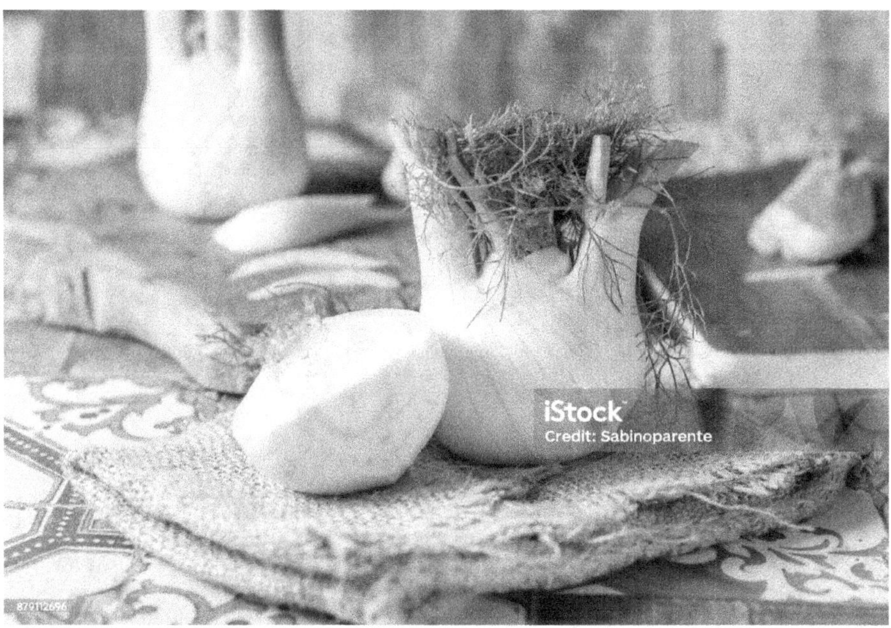

Utilized as a natural remedy for digestive issues, fennel seeds provide numerous benefits to the gastrointestinal tract. The active compounds in fennel, such as anethole and fenchone, help relax the muscles in the gastrointestinal tract, relieving bloating, gas, and heartburn. Fennel also acts as a mild diuretic, promoting urine flow and aiding in the elimination of toxins from the body. Beyond its digestive benefits, fennel seeds possess antimicrobial properties and may help combat harmful bacteria in the gut. Fennel has also been traditionally used as a galactagogue, enhancing breast milk production in nursing mothers. You can enjoy the benefits of fennel by brewing fennel tea or simply chewing on fennel seeds after meals.

4. Chamomile (Matricaria chamomilla):

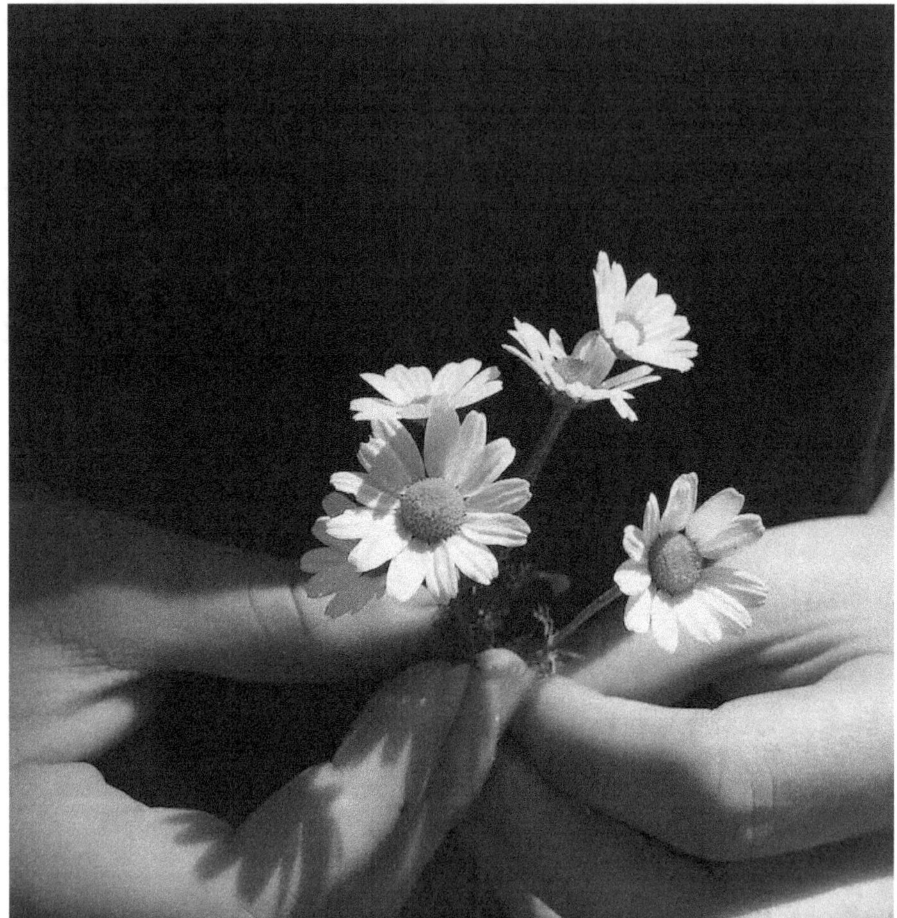

Chamomile offers not only a calming effect but also remarkable digestive support. It contains flavonoids and terpenoids that help relax the smooth muscles in the digestive tract, reducing cramping and promoting healthy digestion. Chamomile is renowned for its gentle sedative properties, aiding in stress relief and improving sleep quality, which can indirectly positively impact digestion. Additionally, chamomile possesses anti-inflammatory and antioxidant properties, which may contribute to its overall health benefits. Chamomile has also demonstrated anxiolytic properties, making it useful in managing symptoms of generalized anxiety disorder. To incorporate chamomile into your routine, you can enjoy a warm cup of chamomile tea after a meal or before bedtime.

5. Licorice (Glycyrrhiza glabra):

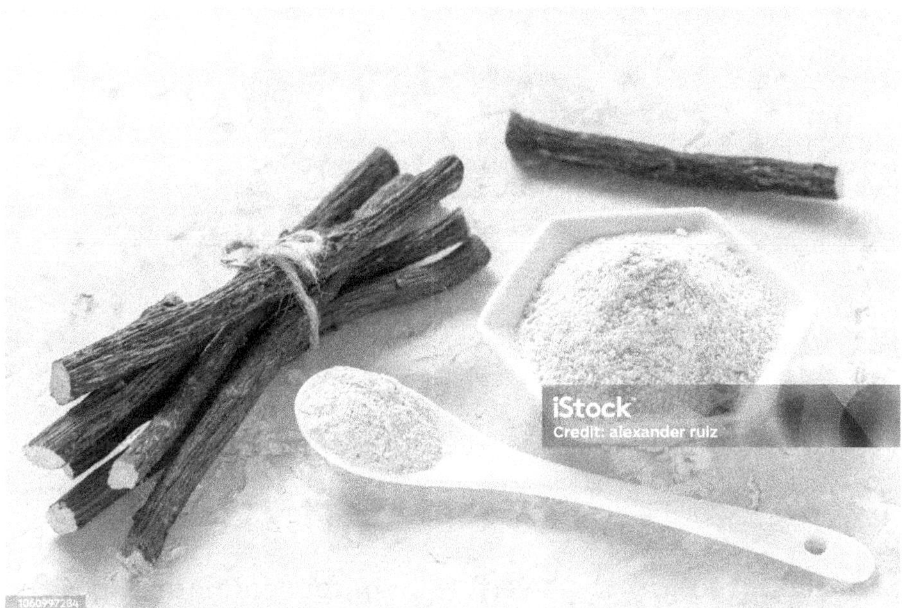

Licorice root has been used for centuries in traditional medicine for its soothing properties on the digestive system. It contains a compound called glycyrrhizin, which helps reduce inflammation in the gastrointestinal tract, relieving symptoms of conditions such as acid reflux and ulcers. Licorice also has an adaptogenic effect, supporting the body's ability to cope with stress. Furthermore, licorice root possesses antimicrobial properties and may aid in balancing gut bacteria. It is important to note that licorice should be used cautiously as it can elevate blood pressure in some individuals. Licorice root has also been studied for its potential anti-viral and anti-inflammatory effects. To enjoy the benefits of licorice, you can brew licorice tea or opt for chewable licorice tablets.

6. Dandelion (Taraxacum officinale):

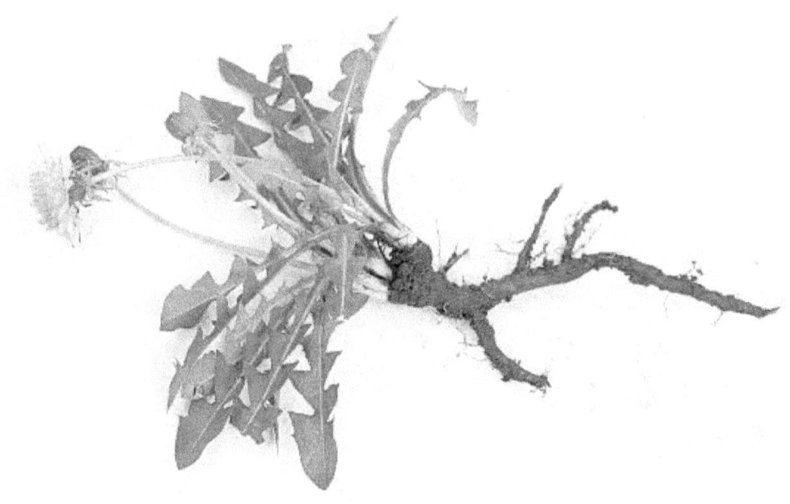

Dandelion root is a powerful herb for promoting healthy digestion. It stimulates the production of bile in the liver, aiding in the breakdown of fats and improving overall digestion. Dandelion root also acts as a gentle laxative, promoting regular bowel movements and relieving constipation. Additionally, dandelion is rich in antioxidants, supporting liver health and detoxification processes in the body. Its diuretic properties have also made it useful in reducing water retention and supporting kidney health. Dandelion root has shown promise in reducing cholesterol levels and managing blood sugar levels. To incorporate dandelion into your routine, you can brew dandelion root tea or take it in capsule form.

7. Marshmallow root (Althaea officinalis):

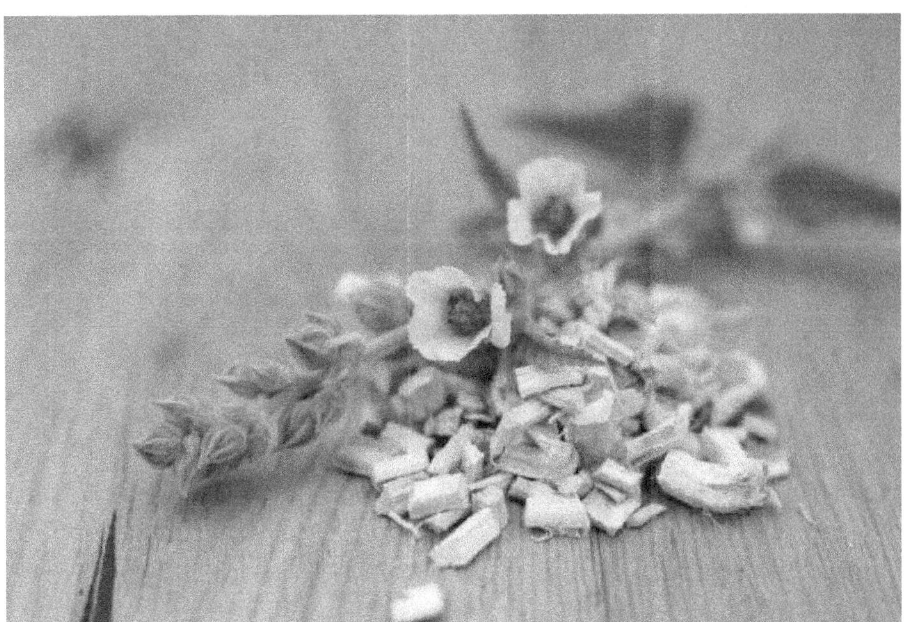

Marshmallow root offers exceptional soothing properties for the digestive system. It contains a mucilage compound that forms a protective layer on the mucous membranes of the gastrointestinal tract, alleviating symptoms of heartburn, indigestion, and irritable bowel syndrome. Marshmallow root also possesses anti-inflammatory properties, further aiding in digestive health. Moreover, marshmallow root may help soothe respiratory issues, such as coughs and sore throats. It has also been traditionally used for its wound-healing properties. You can enjoy the benefits of marshmallow root by brewing it as a tea or taking it in capsule form.

While these herbal remedies can provide relief for digestive issues, it is essential to consult with a healthcare professional before incorporating them into your routine, especially if you have any pre-existing medical conditions or are taking medications. They can provide personalized guidance based on your health history and help monitor any potential interactions.

Incorporating these herbal remedies into your daily routine can help support and maintain a healthy digestive system. However, it is crucial to listen to your body and pay attention to any adverse reactions. If symptoms persist or worsen, it is always best to seek professional medical advice to ensure proper diagnosis and treatment.

In the next chapter, we will explore herbal remedies for stress and anxiety, offering natural solutions for achieving calmness and emotional well-being.

CHAPTER 9
Herbal Remedies for Stress and Anxiety

Stress and anxiety have become increasingly prevalent in today's fast-paced world, affecting individuals from all walks of life. In the quest to find relief, many people have turned to herbal remedies, drawing from the wisdom of traditional healing practices that span centuries. These natural remedies, derived from plants, offer gentle yet effective support to the nervous system, promoting relaxation, calmness, and emotional balance. In this chapter, we delve deeper into the world of herbal remedies for stress and anxiety, uncovering a wider range of herbs and their various applications.

Chamomile, renowned for its soothing properties, takes its place as a cornerstone herb in stress and anxiety management. Its scientific name, Matricaria chamomilla, reflects its maternal nature, as it has been used for centuries to provide comfort and care. Chamomile is rich in flavonoids, which contribute to its calming effects. Not only does it ease anxiety and promote better sleep, but chamomile also offers anti-inflammatory properties that may relieve tension and muscle soreness. Widely recognized for its golden-yellow flowers and apple-like fragrance, chamomile works harmoniously with the nervous system, bringing about relaxation and peace of mind. Often consumed as a warm tea, chamomile can also be found in tincture and essential oil forms, providing alternative methods of administration. Whether sipped slowly or inhaled gently, chamomile's presence can ease restlessness, reduce tension, and foster restorative sleep.

Lavender, aromatic and versatile, emerges as another powerful herbal ally that accompanies individuals on their journey toward stress and anxiety reduction. Lavandula angustifolia, commonly known as lavender, has a long history of therapeutic use. With delicate purple flowers and palming scent, lavender possesses profound soothing effects on the mind and body. Lavender contains linalool and linalyl acetate, chemicals that promote relaxation and reduce feelings of stress and anxiety. Recognized for its timeless association with relaxation, the dried flowers of lavender can be used to create herbal sachets that release their therapeutic aroma when placed beneath pillows or carried in pockets. Additionally, lavender essential oil, when inhaled or diffused, initiates a cascade of tranquility, melting away anxiety and promoting a sense of serenity within.

Among the herbs recommended for stress and anxiety relief, lemon balm finds its rightful place as a gentle yet potent option for those seeking emotional balance and calm. Melissa officinalis, commonly known as lemon balm, derives its name from the Greek word for "honeybee" due to its alluring scent. This vibrant and citrus-scented herb has long been utilized in traditional medicine for its anxiolytic properties. Lemon balm contains rosmarinic acid, a compound that helps regulate GABA receptors in the brain, promoting relaxation and reducing anxiety. Lemon balm elicits a gentle calming effect on the nervous system, helping to reduce anxiety, ease restlessness, and enhance cognitive function. Preparations of lemon balm as a tea, often combined with other soothing herbs like chamomile or passionflower, or as a tincture, have been embraced by many individuals seeking solace from the overwhelming pressures of daily life.

Passionflower,

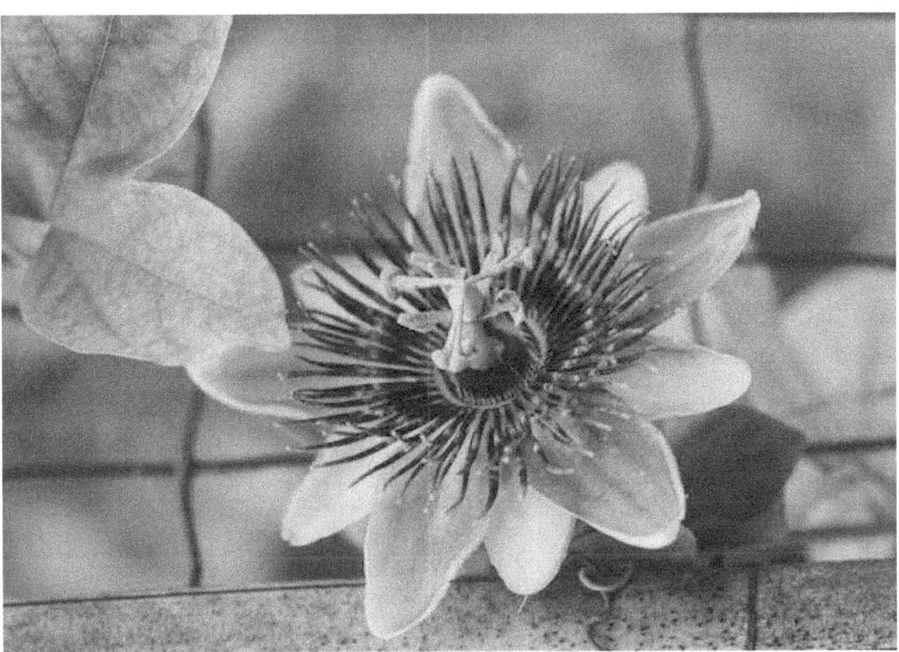

revered for its exquisite and captivating blooms, unfurls as a potent herb that embodies serenity and tranquility. The scientific name Passiflora incarnata reveals its spiritual and symbolic association with the Passion of Christ, emphasizing its calming and restorative qualities. Passionflower contains flavonoids and alkaloids such as harmine, which enhance the production of gamma-aminobutyric acid (GABA) in the brain, resulting in a sedative and anxiolytic effect. Rich in compounds that interact with the brain's receptors, passionflower has been prized in traditional herbal medicine for its ability to calm nervousness and alleviate anxiety. This herb is often consumed as a tea or tincture, allowing its delicate flavor and essence to gradually invite relaxation. Passionflower may also be found in combination formulas with other calming herbs to enhance its effects. It is important to note that passionflower may cause drowsiness, making it most suitable for evening consumption or during times when relaxation and unwinding are desired.

Beyond these well-known herbs, an array of stunning botanical allies step forward, offering their unique strengths in the battle against stress and anxiety. Ashwagandha (Withania somnifera), revered in Ayurvedic medicine, holds adaptogenic properties that strengthen the body's response to stress by supporting the adrenal glands. Ashwagandha, often referred to as the "Indian Ginseng," helps stabilize cortisol levels, promotes mental clarity, and balances energy levels. With its ancient roots deeply entwined in Ayurveda, it has been trusted for centuries as a natural remedy for stress and anxiety. Its root is commonly used in powdered form and incorporated into beverages and recipes. Regular consumption of ashwagandha may help reduce stress-related symptoms, boost overall well-being, and enhance resilience in challenging times.

Valerian root (Valeriana officinalis), a perennial herb with a pungent aroma, aids in promoting relaxation and restful sleep. Valerenic acid and valtrates found in the root of the valerian plant have been shown to enhance the availability and function of GABA, thus reducing anxiety and promoting calmness. Valerian root has been trusted for centuries as a natural sedative and is often consumed as a tea or in tincture form. It may take time for the effects to fully manifest, so consistent use is key for those seeking its benefits. Although valerian root is generally safe, it is advisable to exercise caution, especially when combining it with other sedatives or medications that affect the central nervous system.

Skullcap (Scutellaria lateriflora),

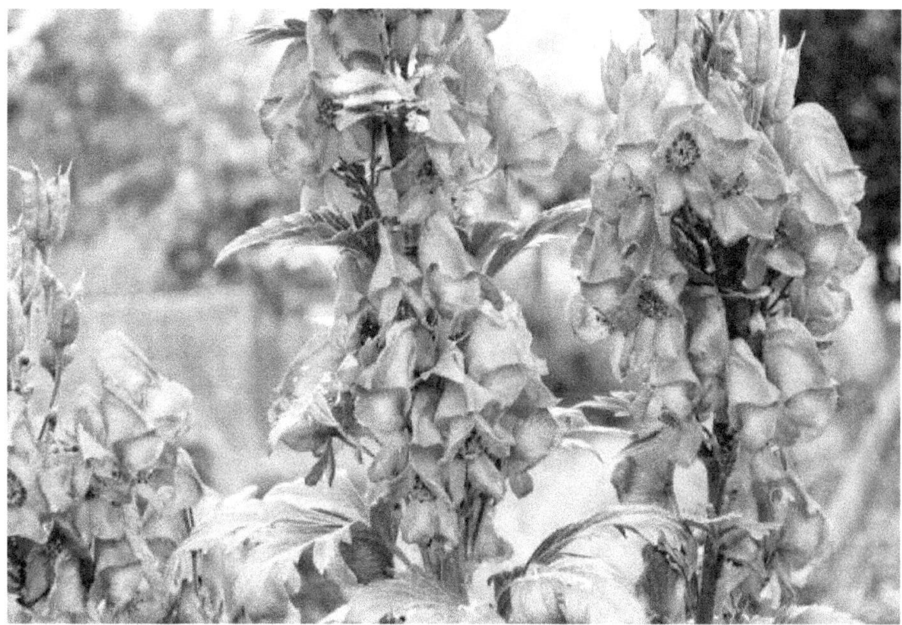

a delicate flowering herb, has a long history of use in traditional Native American and Western herbal medicine for its calming effects on the nervous system. Skullcap contains flavonoids such as baicalin, which possess anxiolytic properties and help reduce anxiety and stress. This herb is often used to alleviate tension and anxiety, promote relaxation, and support restful sleep. Skullcap can be consumed as tea or tincture and is sometimes combined with other calming herbs, such as chamomile or lemon balm, for enhanced effects. Its gentle nature makes it suitable for regular use during times of increased stress or emotional turmoil.

Lastly, **holy basil (Ocimum sanctum),**

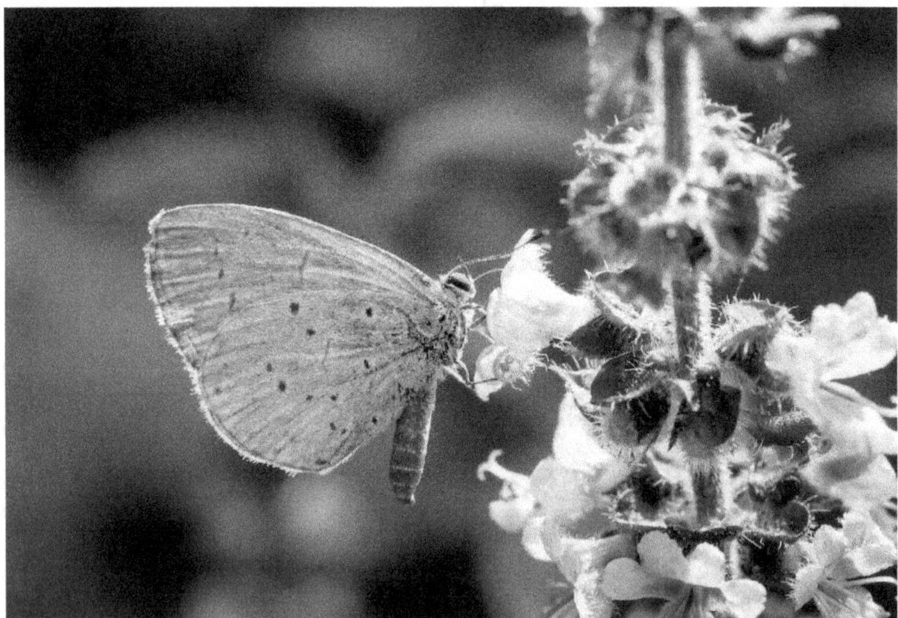

considered sacred in Indian traditions, serves as an adaptogenic herb that helps the mind and body adapt to stress. Also known as tulsi, holy basil has been treasured for its medicinal properties for thousands of years. Holy basil contains eugenol, rosmarinic acid, and other compounds that possess anti-inflammatory and anti-anxiety properties, helping to alleviate stress and promote relaxation. Its leaves can be brewed into tea or taken as a tincture to support overall well-being during challenging times. Holy basil also exhibits immune-boosting effects, making it a valuable addition to one's stress management routine.

It is crucial to remember that when using herbal remedies for stress and anxiety, individual responses may vary. Consulting with a qualified healthcare practitioner or herbalist is highly recommended, especially for those currently taking medications or managing underlying conditions. It is important to disclose any current medications, medical history, or allergies to ensure the safe and effective usage of herbal remedies.

Additionally, it is important to note that herbal remedies can take time to work, and consistency is key. Building a daily routine that incorporates herbal remedies, along with other stress management techniques like mindfulness, exercise, and healthy lifestyle choices, can yield the best results.

Herbal remedies offer a natural and holistic approach to managing stress and anxiety. Chamomile, lavender, lemon balm, passionflower, ashwagandha, valerian root, skullcap, and holy basil are just a few examples of the vast array of herbs that can support the nervous system, promote relaxation, and enhance emotional well-being. By harnessing the power of nature, individuals can find solace and relief from the burdensome effects of stress and anxiety. Coupled with self-care practices and professional guidance, these herbal allies can form an integral part of a comprehensive approach to managing and reducing stress in daily life.

CHAPTER 10
Herbal Remedies for Skin Care

Our skin, the largest organ of our body, requires special care and nourishment to stay healthy and radiant. While there are countless skincare products available in the market, sometimes the best solutions can be found in nature. Herbal remedies offer a holistic approach to skincare, harnessing the power of plants to rejuvenate, heal, and enhance the health of our skin. In this chapter, we will explore an extended list of herbal remedies, each with their unique benefits, for achieving optimal skin health.

1. Aloe Vera:

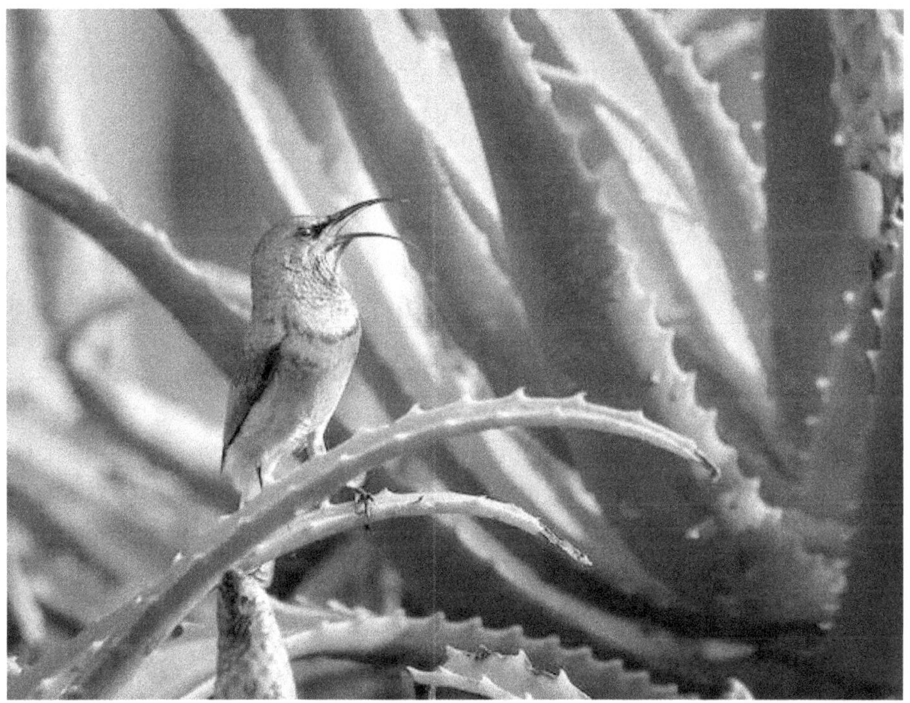

Known as the "plant of immortality, "aloe vera has been used for centuries to treat various skin ailments. Its gel, extracted from the succulent leaves, possesses remarkable healing properties. Aloe vera gel can soothe sunburns, reduce inflammation, and moisturize the skin. It contains enzymes that stimulate the production of collagen, promoting skin elasticity and reducing the appearance of wrinkles. Aloe vera gel can also aid in the treatment of acne due to its antimicrobial properties.

2.　　**Calendula:** Calendula, also referred to as marigold, has been used for centuries as a healing herb. Its vibrant flowers contain anti-inflammatory and antibacterial compounds that make it ideal for soothing and repairing damaged skin. Calendula oil or cream can be applied topically to treat skin conditions such as eczema, dermatitis, and dryness. It has also been found to support wound healing and reduce the formation of scar tissue.

3.   **Chamomile:** Chamomile, with its small daisy-like flowers, has long been valued for its calming and anti-inflammatory properties. It can soothe irritated or sensitive skin, reduce redness, and alleviate conditions like rosacea and eczema. Chamomile tea, when used as a facial steam, can promote deep pore cleansing and gentle exfoliation. Additionally, chamomile extract can be added to skincare products to provide a soothing effect and reduce skin irritation.

4.   **Lavender:** Lavender, known for its beautiful purple flowers and delightful fragrance, offers a multitude of benefits for the skin. Its essential oil possesses antimicrobial, anti-inflammatory, and antioxidant properties, making it effective in treating acne, reducing inflammation, and promoting overall skin health. Lavender oil can also be used as a calming agent, helping to relax the mind and alleviate stress. Diluted lavender oil can be applied topically or added to bathwater for a rejuvenating and aromatic experience.

5. **Rosemary:**

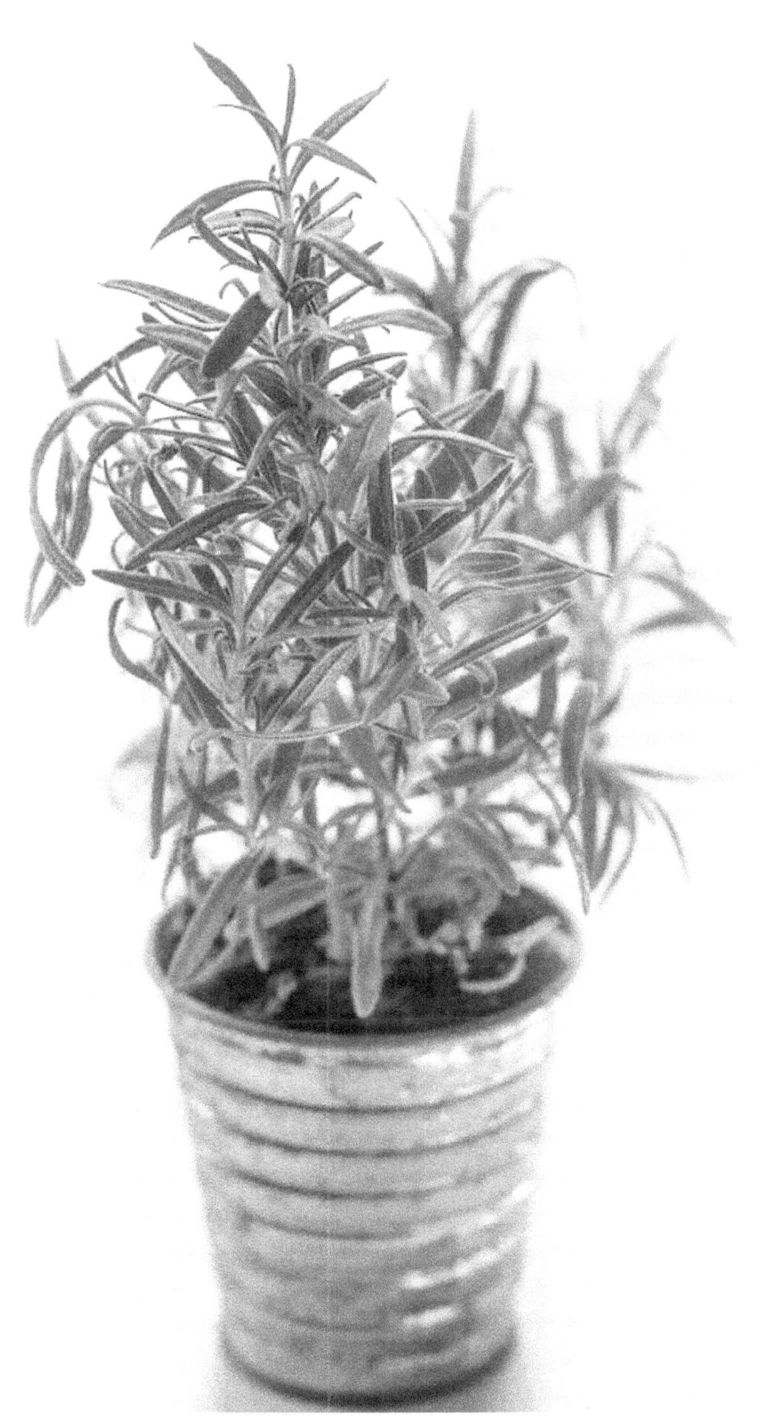

This versatile herb not only adds flavor to our culinary creations but also offers benefits for our skin. Rosemary possesses powerful antioxidant properties, protecting the skin from environmental damage and premature aging. Its stimulating effect on circulation promotes a healthy complexion while reducing puffiness and under-eye bags. Rosemary essential oil can be blended with carrier oils and applied topically or used in homemade face masks to invigorate and rejuvenate the skin.

6. **Turmeric**: Widely used in traditional Ayurvedic medicine, turmeric is a potent herb with numerous benefits for the skin. Curcumin, its active compound, possesses anti-inflammatory, antioxidant, and antimicrobial properties. Turmeric can help combat acne, reduce redness, and brighten the skin. Its healing properties make it useful in treating scars, hyperpigmentation, and other skin conditions. A turmeric paste or mask can be applied topically to achieve these benefits. However, it is important to note that turmeric can temporarily stain the skin, so care should be taken while using it.

7. **Witch Hazel:**

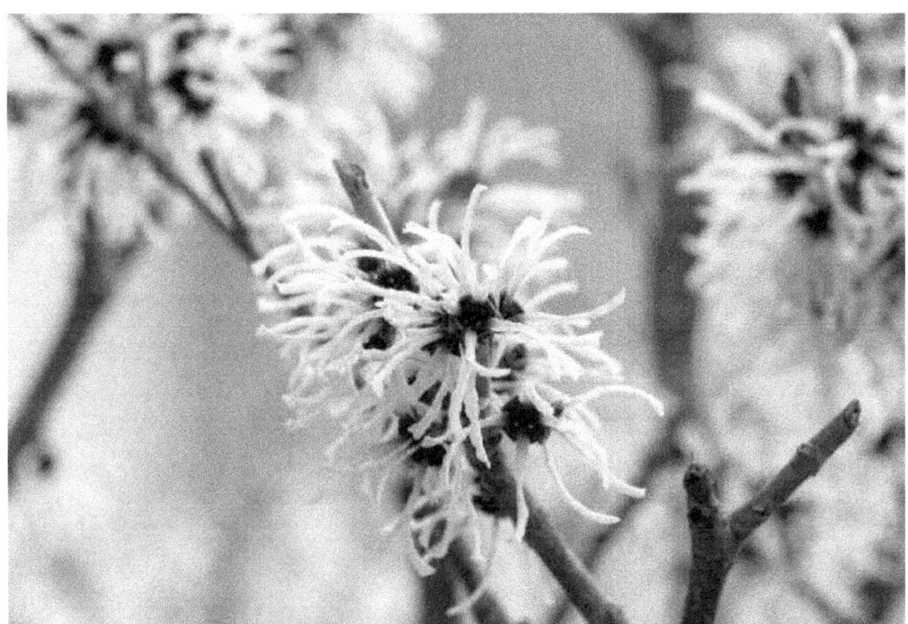

Witch hazel, derived from the bark and leaves of the witch hazel plant, has been used for centuries as a natural astringent. It helps tighten the skin, reduce the appearance of pores, and regulate oil production, making it particularly beneficial for oily or acne-prone skin. Witch hazel also possesses anti-inflammatory properties, making it effective in soothing skin irritations such as insect bites, rashes, and sunburns. Witch hazel distillate can be applied directly to the skin or incorporated into homemade toners and cleansers.

8. Jojoba Oil:

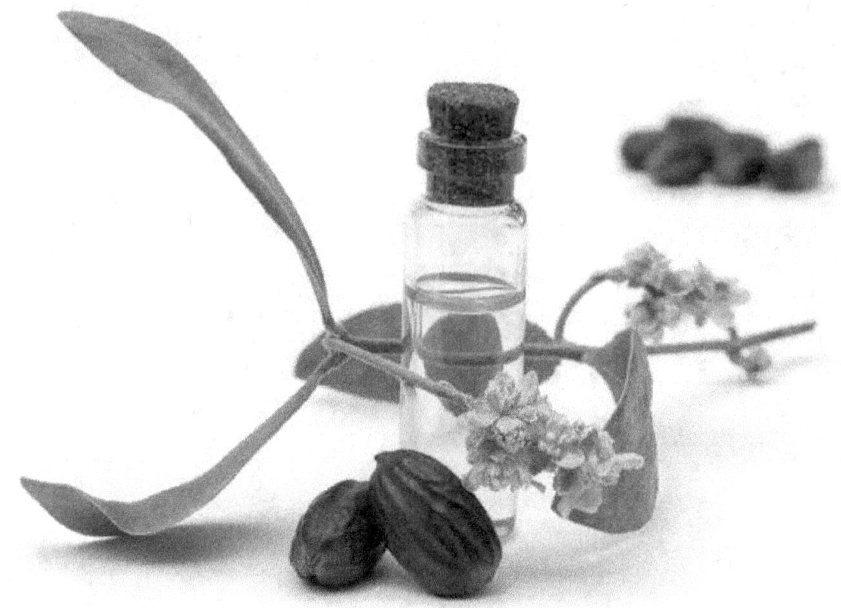

Despite being referred to as an oil, jojoba oil is a liquid wax that closely resembles the sebum our skin produces naturally. This unique characteristic makes it an excellent moisturizer that can balance oil production, maintain the skin barrier, and minimize moisture loss. Jojoba oil is easily absorbed, non-comedogenic, and suitable for all skin types. Its nourishing properties make it effective in reducing the appearance of fine lines and wrinkles, promoting a healthy complexion and a youthful glow.

9. Tea Tree Oil:

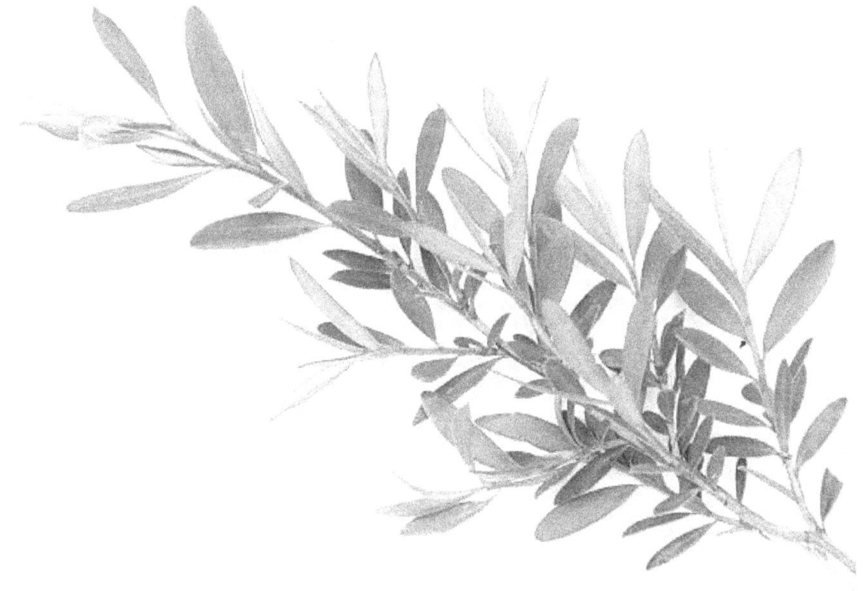

Tea tree oil, derived from the leaves of the tea tree plant, possesses powerful antimicrobial and anti-inflammatory properties. It is well-known for its effectiveness in combating acne and other skin infections. Tea tree oil can penetrate the skin's pores, unclogging them and reducing the growth of acne-causing bacteria. However, caution should be exercised while using tea tree oil, as it can be harsh and dry to the skin when used undiluted. It is recommended to dilute tea tree oil with carrier oil or add it to skincare products in appropriate concentrations.

10. Oatmeal:

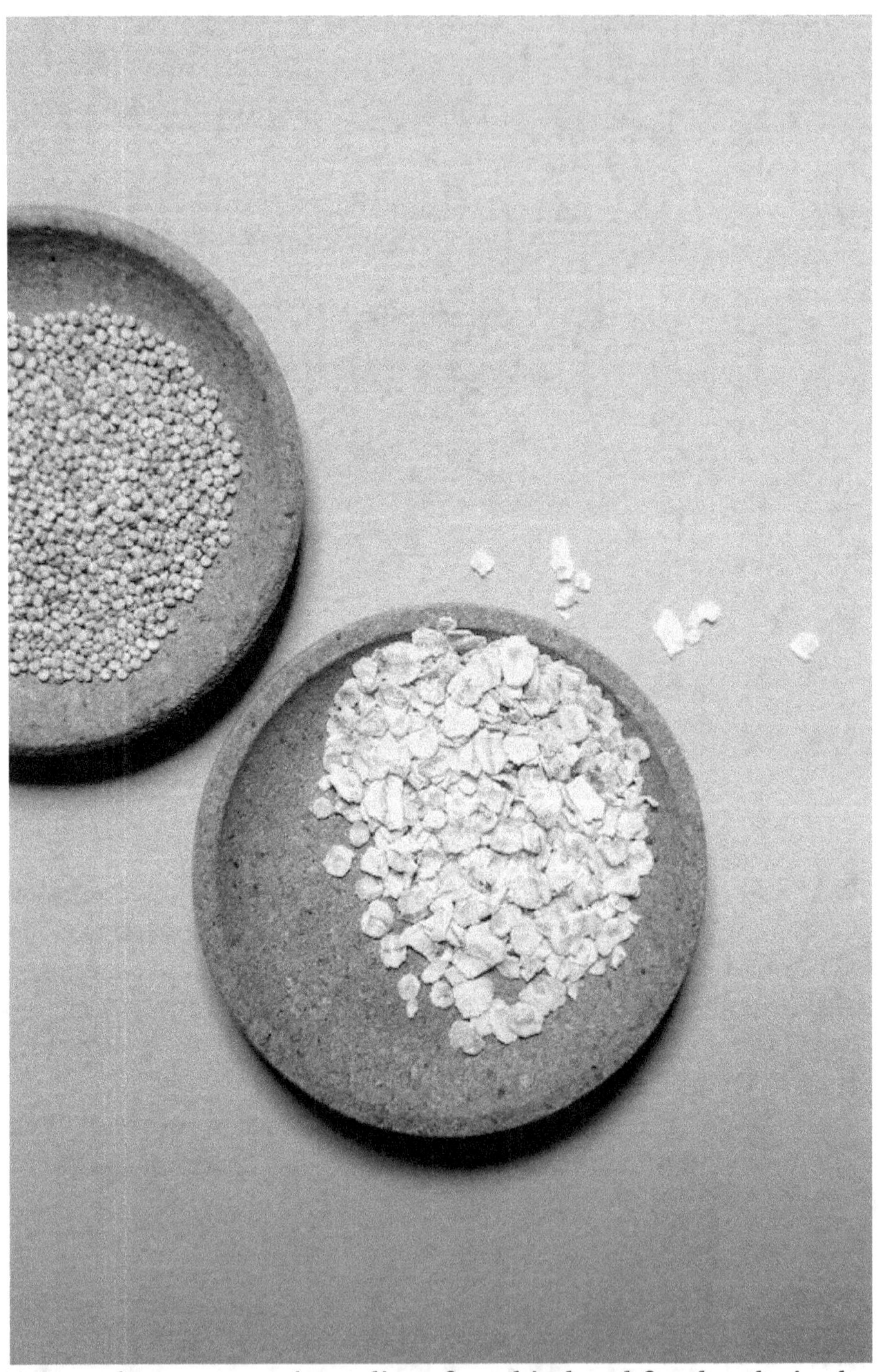

Oatmeal, a common ingredient found in breakfast bowls, is also a gentle and effective treatment for various skin conditions. It contains natural substances such as beta-glucans and phenols that possess anti-inflammatory, moisturizing, and soothing properties. Oatmeal helps to relieve itching, redness, and dryness associated with conditions like eczema, psoriasis, and sunburn. It can be used as an ingredient in homemade face masks, baths, or body scrubs to nourish and calm the skin. Colloidal oatmeal, which is finely ground oatmeal, is particularly suited for skincare applications.

These herbal remedies present a natural and holistic approach to skincare, catering to different skin types and concerns. It is important to note that while these remedies are generally safe, it is advisable to perform a patch test before applying them to a larger area of the skin, especially for those with sensitive skin or known allergies. Additionally, for individuals with existing skin conditions or concerns, consulting with a dermatologist or herbalist is recommended.

By incorporating these herbal remedies into your skincare routine, you can harness the power of nature to achieve healthy, radiant skin. Embrace the beauty and healing properties of these herbs, and let your skin glow with natural vitality.

CHAPTER 11
<u>Herbal Remedies for Women's Health</u>

Women's health is a complex and multifaceted aspect of well-being, requiring special attention and care. Throughout history, herbal remedies have played an essential role in supporting women's health at different stages of life. From menstrual concerns to reproductive health and menopause, nature offers an array of plants that can provide relief and promote balance.

1. Menstrual Health:

Women often face various challenges during their menstrual cycle, such as cramps, irregular periods, and bloating. Herbal remedies can offer gentle and effective support in managing these symptoms. Some commonly used herbs for menstrual health include:

- Chasteberry (Vitex agnus-castus):

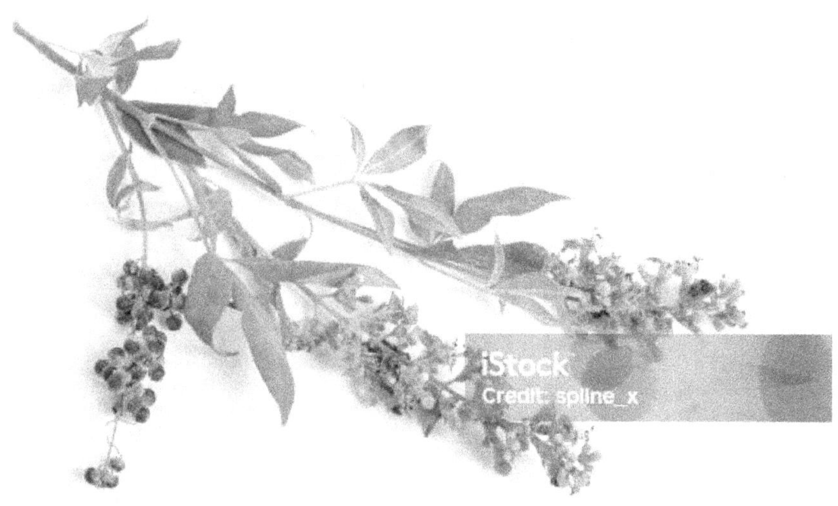

This herb helps regulate hormones and balance the menstrual cycle, making it useful for irregular periods and premenstrual syndrome (PMS). Chasteberry acts on the pituitary gland, promoting a balance between estrogen and progesterone levels, thereby alleviating common menstrual symptoms. It can also be beneficial for women with conditions such as endometriosis or fibroid.

-

- **Cramp bark (Viburnum opulus):**

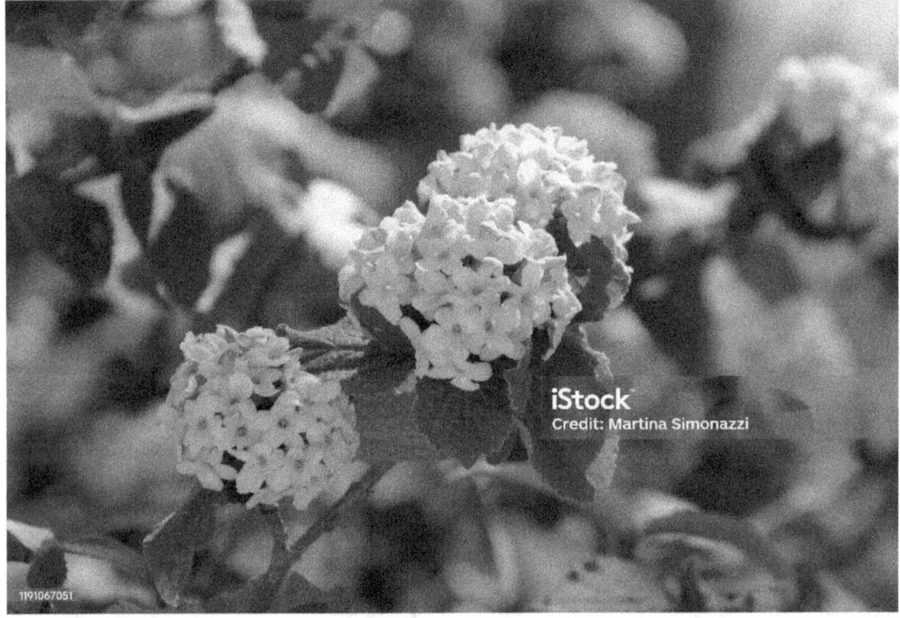

As the name suggests, cramp bark can alleviate menstrual cramps by relaxing the uterine muscles. It contains antispasmodic compounds that help reduce muscular tension and relieve pain. This herb is particularly beneficial for women who experience painful cramps during menstruation. Cramp bark can also be helpful for women with conditions like uterine fibroid or ovarian cyst.

- **Red raspberry leaf (Rubus idaeus):**

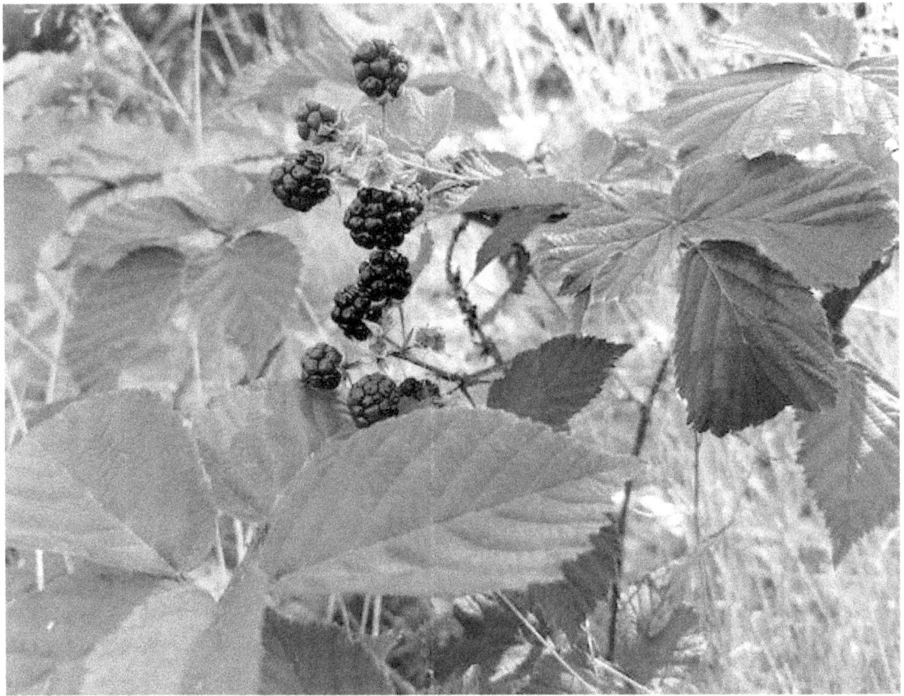

Rich in nutrients, red raspberry leaf can tone the uterus and ease excessive menstrual bleeding. It contains compounds that help strengthen and relax the muscles of the uterus. Additionally, red raspberry leaf is known to support overall reproductive health and may be helpful for women trying to conceive. It is also a valuable herb during pregnancy, aiding in the preparation of the uterus and promoting smooth labor.

2. Reproductive Health:

Maintaining reproductive health is crucial for women, especially when planning for conception or addressing issues like hormonal imbalances or polycystic ovary syndrome (PCOS). Herbal remedies that support reproductive health Include **Dong Quai (Angelica sinensis):**

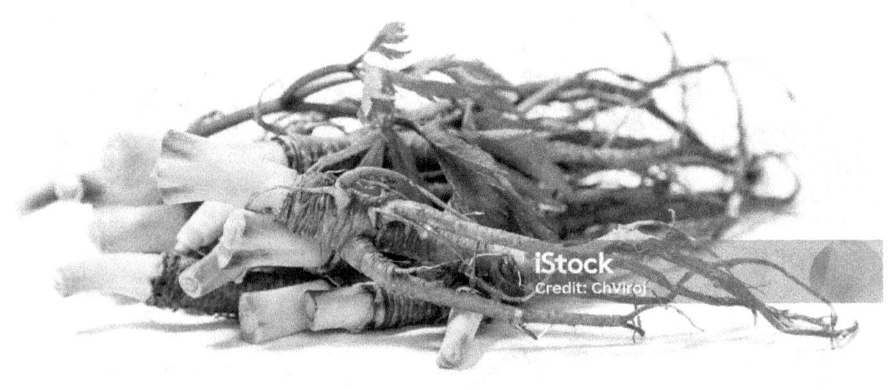

Dong Quai is widely used in traditional Chinese medicine to balance hormones, regulate the menstrual cycle, and support fertility. It contains phytoestrogens that can have a regulating effect on hormonal activity and may help improve reproductive function. It is particularly beneficial for women experiencing menstrual irregularities or dealing with symptoms of hormonal imbalance. Dong Quai should be used cautiously by women with heavy periods or those taking blood-thinning medications.

- Black cohosh (Actaea racemosa):

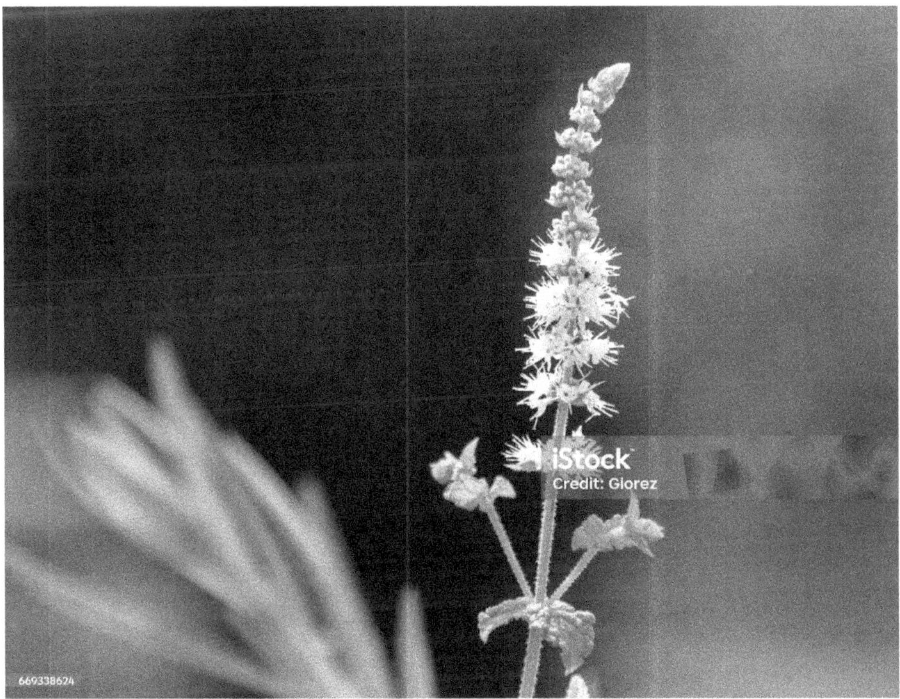

This herb is known for its ability to relieve menopausal symptoms, but it can also help with menstrual irregularities and support hormonal balance. Black cohosh contains compounds that act as estrogen-like substances in the body, helping to restore balance during various reproductive stages. It may be particularly useful for women experiencing early menopausal symptoms or menstrual disturbances. However, black cohosh should be avoided by women with liver conditions and used under the guidance of a healthcare professional.

- Vitex (Vitex agnus-castus):

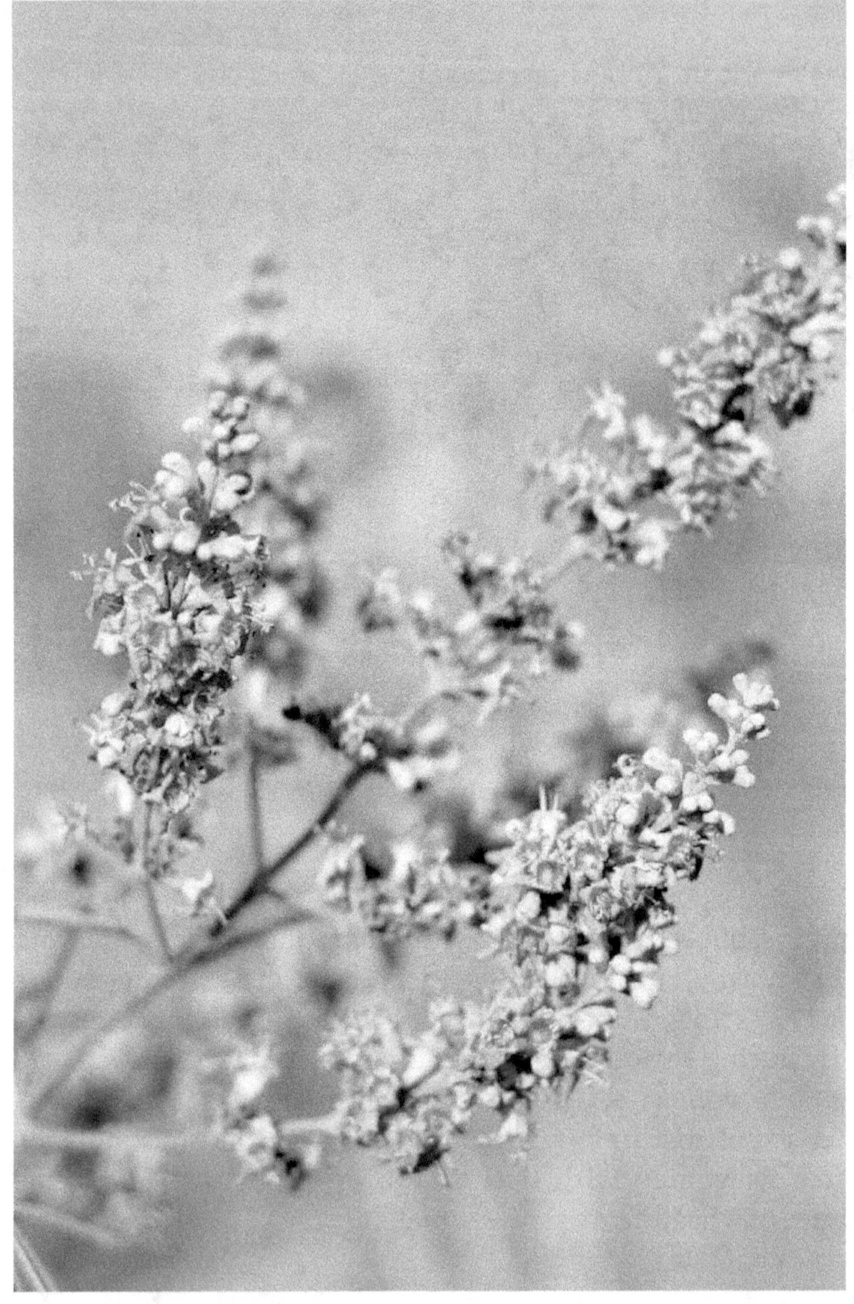

As mentioned earlier, Vitex is beneficial for reproductive health, promoting ovulation and regulating the menstrual cycle. It acts on the hypothalamic-pituitary-ovarian axis, thereby balancing hormone production and improving fertility. Vitex is often used in cases of irregular periods, premenstrual syndrome (PMS), and even for supporting fertility in women with certain ovulatory disorders. It should not be used during pregnancy.

3. Menopausal Support:

Menopause is a natural phase in a woman's life, but it can bring uncomfortable symptoms like hot flashes, mood changes, and insomnia. Herbal remedies can help alleviate these symptoms and support overall well-being:

- Black cohosh (Actaea racemosa):

As one of the most well-known herbs for menopause, black cohosh can reduce hot flashes and night sweats while supporting hormonal balance. Its phytoestrogenic compounds can compensate for the decline in estrogen levels during menopause, helping to reduce the frequency and intensity of hot flashes and other related symptoms. It may also help improve sleep quality and reduce anxiety associated with menopause.

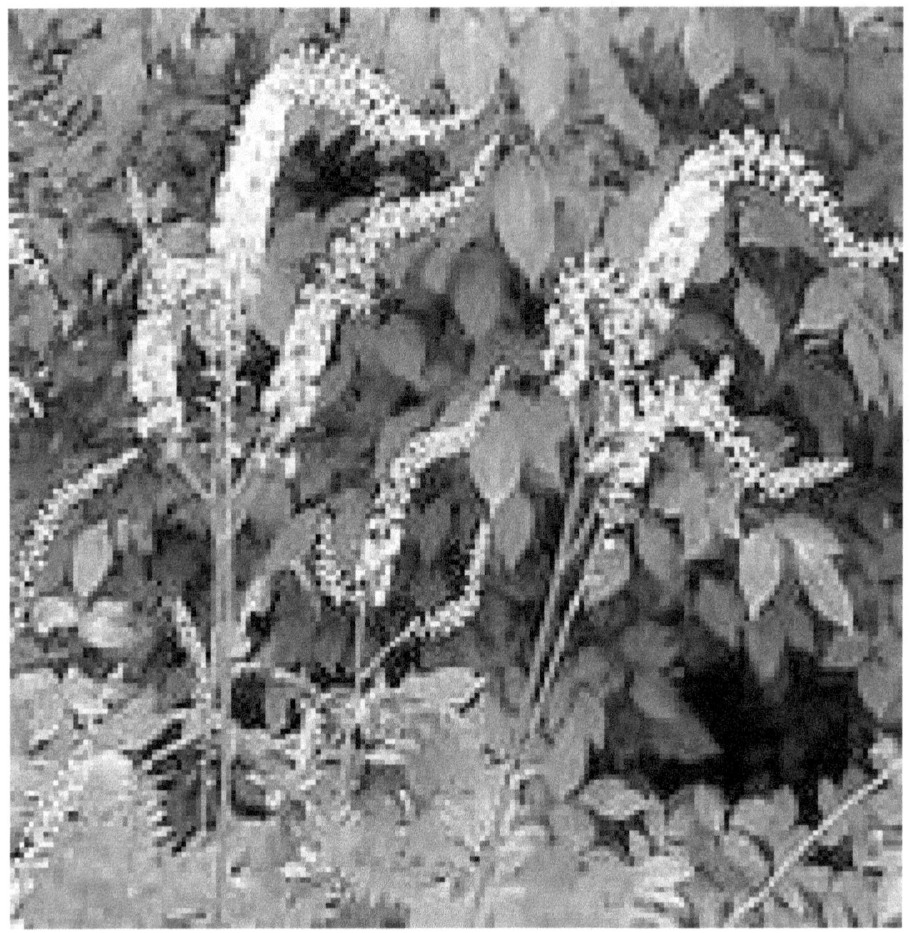

- St. John's Wort (Hypericum perforatum):
This herb is widely used for mood support and can be beneficial for managing mood swings and mild depression during menopause. St. John's Wort contains hypericin and other compounds that act as natural serotonin reuptake inhibitors, potentially helping to stabilize mood and improve overall well-being during this transitional phase. However, St. John's Wort may interact with certain medications, so it's essential to consult with a healthcare professional before use.

- Sage (Salvia officinalis):

Known for its cooling properties, sage can ease hot flashes, night sweats, and excessive sweating. It contains compounds that help regulate body temperature and reduce the intensity of vasomotor symptoms associated with menopause. Sage can be used both internally as a tea or tincture and externally as a topical remedy for night sweats. It is also known to support memory and cognitive function, which can be beneficial during menopausal periods of mental fog and forgetfulness.

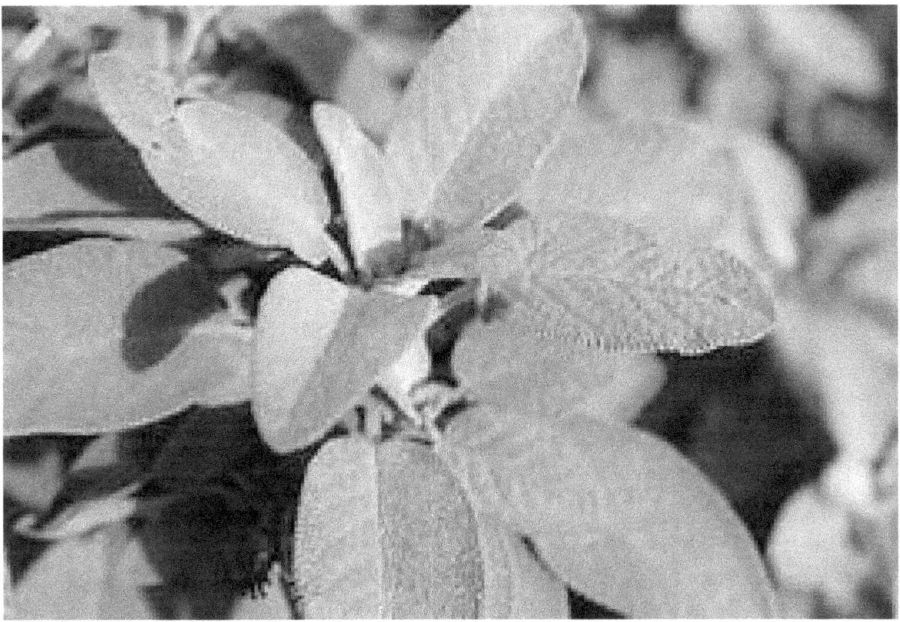

It's important to consult with a healthcare professional or herbalist before using herbal remedies, especially if you have any underlying health conditions or are taking medications. While herbal remedies can offer valuable support, individual needs and responses may vary. Embracing a holistic approach to women's health involves self-care, proper nutrition, regular exercise, and mindfulness along with incorporating sage herbal remedies into your routine. By respecting and nurturing your body's natural rhythms, you can find balance and vitality throughout every stage of womanhood.

CHAPTER 12
Herbal Remedies for Boosting Immunity

In today's fast-paced and stressful world, maintaining a strong immune system is crucial for overall health and well-being. While there are many factors that contribute to a healthy immune system, incorporating herbal remedies into your daily routine can provide a natural boost to your body's defenses (Schwarb, et al. 2023).

1. Echinacea (Echinacea purpurea):

Echinacea is one of the most popular herbs known for its immune-boosting properties. It has been used for centuries by Native Americans as a remedy for various ailments. Echinacea stimulates the production of white blood cells, which play a vital role in fighting off infections. It contains a variety of active compounds, including alkylamides, polysaccharides, and flavonoids, which have been shown to enhance immune function.

Research suggests that Echinacea may reduce the risk and duration of upper respiratory tract infections, such as the common cold. It activates immune cells, promotes the release of cytokines, and increases the activity of natural killer cells. Additionally, Echinacea has anti-inflammatory and antioxidant properties, further supporting immune health. Echinacea can be consumed as a tea, tincture, or in capsule form.

Elderberry (Sambucus nigra):

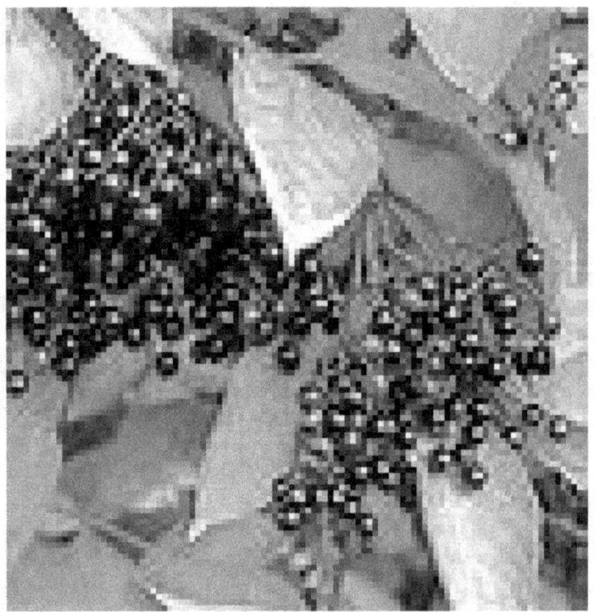

Elderberry is another herb widely recognized for its ability to enhance immune function. The dark purple berries of the elderberry plant are rich in antioxidants and have been used for centuries to support the immune system. Elderberry contains high levels of vitamin C and other immune-boosting compounds, such as anthocyanins, that help to reduce the duration and severity of cold and flu symptoms.

Clinical trials have demonstrated the effectiveness of elderberry in reducing the duration of cold and flu symptoms by inhibiting their application of the immune response. Elderberry has also shown anti-inflammatory properties, reducing congestion and improving overall respiratory health. Elderberry can be consumed as a syrup, tea, or in supplement form.

2. **stragalus (Astragalus membranaceus):**

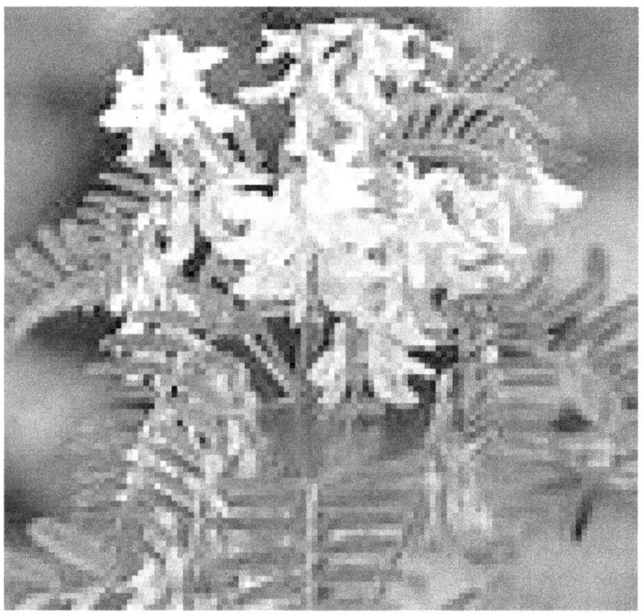

Astragalus is an herb that has been used in Traditional Chinese Medicine for centuries for its immune-enhancing properties. It is known as an adaptogen, which means it helps the body adapt to stress and supports overall well-being.

Astragalus contains polysaccharides and saponins that have been shown to increase the activity of immune cells, such as T cells and natural killer cells, and enhance their ability to recognize and destroy pathogens. It may also have anti-inflammatory effects, promoting a balanced immune response.

Incorporating astragalus into your daily routine may help reduce the frequency and severity of respiratory infections and support overall immune health. Astragalus can be consumed as a tea, tincture, or in capsule form. It is important to note that individuals with autoimmune diseases or those taking immunosuppressive medications should consult with a healthcare professional before using astragalus.

3. Garlic (Allium sativum):

Garlic is a powerful immune booster with antimicrobial and antiviral properties. It has been used for centuries in various cultures for its medicinal properties. Garlic contains compounds, including allicin, that help stimulate the production and activity of immune cells, such as macrophages and lymphocytes. Allicin also exhibits antioxidant effects, protecting immune cells from oxidative damage.

Many studies have indicated that regular consumption of garlic may enhance immune function, reduce the risk of respiratory infections, and decrease the duration of illnesses. Garlic's antimicrobial properties make it a valuable ally in combating pathogens. Incorporating fresh garlic into your meals or taking garlic supplements can provide immune support.

4. Turmeric (Curcuma longa):

Turmeric is a vibrant yellow spice widely recognized for its numerous health benefits, including immune support. It contains a compound called curcumin, which has been extensively studied for its immunomodulatory effects. Curcumin exhibits antioxidant and anti-inflammatory properties, helping to reduce inflammation and oxidative stress, which are crucial factors in maintaining a balanced immune system.

Research suggests that curcumin can support immune cell activity and modulate immune responses (Rubegeta, et al. 2023). It may enhance the production of antibodies, stimulate the activity of natural killer cells, and regulate the release of immune signaling molecules. Turmeric can be used in cooking or consumed as a supplement. To enhance its absorption, it is recommended to consume turmeric with black pepper or in liposomal form.

5. Ginger (Zingiber officinale):

Ginger is a versatile herb known for its warming and immune-boosting properties. It has been used traditionally to alleviate symptoms of respiratory infections and strengthen the body's defense mechanisms. Ginger contains gingerol, a bioactive compound with antimicrobial and anti-inflammatory effects.

Studies have shown that ginger exhibits immunomodulatory effects by enhancing the activity of immune cells, such as T cells and natural killer cells, and reducing pro-inflammatory cytokines. Ginger also supports respiratory health and helps to clear congestion. Drinking ginger tea or adding fresh ginger to your meals can provide immune support and soothe symptoms during illnesses.

6. Reishi Mushroom (Ganoderma lucidum):

Reishi mushroom is a revered herb in Traditional Chinese Medicine known for its immune-modulating properties. It helps to balance and strengthen the immune system, making it more effective in fighting off infections. Reishi mushroom contains beta-glucans, triterpenes, and polysaccharides that have been shown to enhance immune function.

Research has demonstrated that Reishi mushroom can increase the activity of natural killer cells, enhance antibody production, and stimulate the release of immune-modulating compounds. It may also have anti-inflammatory effects, supporting a balanced immune response. Reishi mushroom can be consumed as a tea, tincture, or in powder form. Consult with a healthcare professional if you have bleeding disorders, low blood pressure, or are taking immunosuppressive medications before using Reishi mushroom.

7. Holy Basil (Ocimum sanctum):

Holy basil, also known as Tulsi, is an adaptogenic herb that supports immune function by reducing stress and inflammation. It has been highly regarded in Ayurvedic medicine for its ability to promote longevity, vitality, and overall health. Holy basil contains eugenol, rosmarinic acid, and other bioactive compounds that contribute to its immune-boosting properties.

Studies have shown that holy basil exhibits antioxidant and immunomodulatory effects by enhancing the activity of immune cells, reducing oxidative stress, and regulating immune responses. It also helps to balance cortisol levels, a stress hormone that can compromise immune function when elevated for prolonged periods. Consuming holy basil as a tea or incorporating it into your daily routine through supplements can provide immune support.

It's important to note that while herbal remedies can provide support for the immune system, they should not replace a healthy lifestyle and medical advice. It's always recommended to consult with a healthcare professional before starting any new herbal regimen, especially if you have underlying health conditions or are taking medications.

Incorporating these herbal remedies into your daily routine can help strengthen your immune system and improve your overall health. Remember to choose high-quality herbs and use them responsibly to harness their full potential. Embrace the power of nature and give your immune system the support it needs to thrive.

CHAPTER 13
Herbal Remedies for Respiratory Health

Respiratory health plays a crucial role in our overall well-being. Breathing freely and easily allows us to engage in daily activities without limitations. However, respiratory issues such as congestion, cough, allergies, and infections can disrupt our lives and cause discomfort. Fortunately, herbal remedies have been used for centuries to alleviate respiratory symptoms and promote respiratory health. In this chapter, we will explore several powerful herbs that can help improve your respiratory health (Schwarb, et al. 2023).

1. **Eucalyptus (Eucalyptus globulus):**

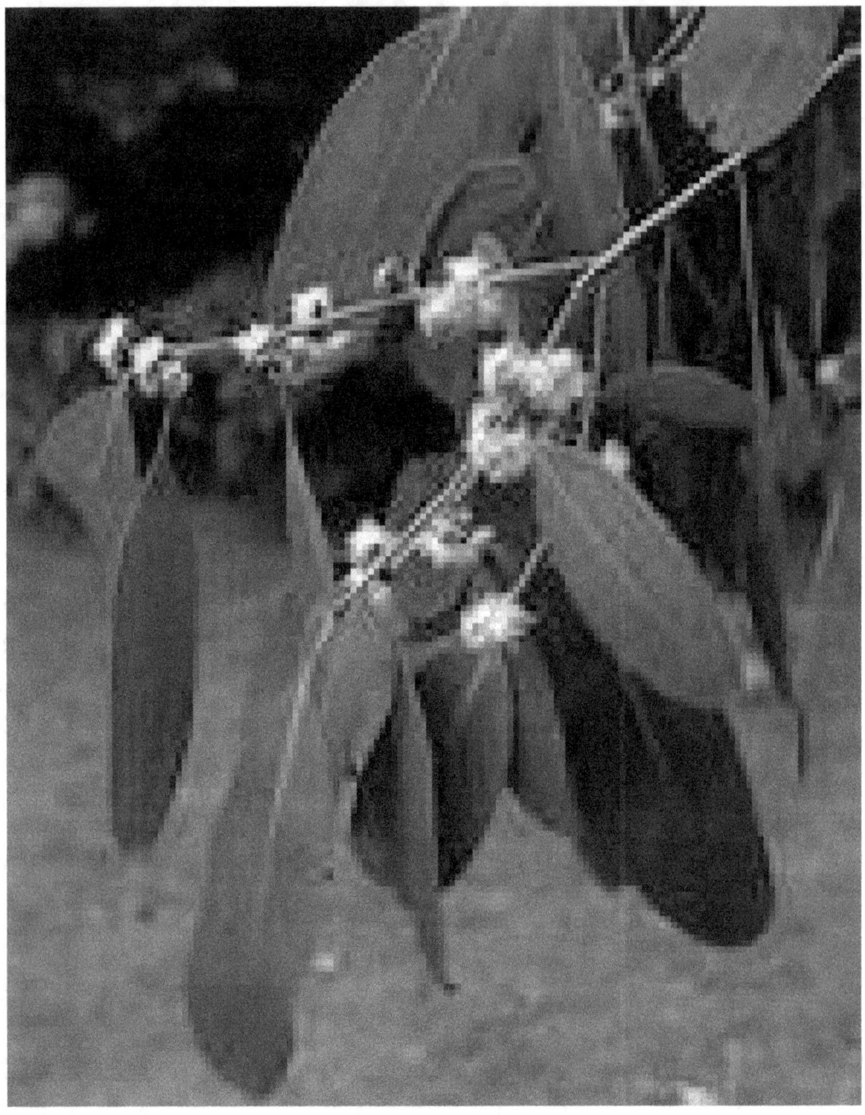

Known for its refreshing fragrance, eucalyptus is highly effective in treating respiratory conditions. The essential oil of eucalyptus contains compounds called cineole, which have expectorant and decongestant properties. Inhaling steam infused with eucalyptus oil can help clear nasal passages and relieve coughs. It can also soothe sore throats and ease breathing difficulties. Eucalyptus can be found in various forms, including essential oils, lozenges, and chest rubs. Additionally, eucalyptus essential oil can be applied topically to the chest and back to provide further relief from respiratory symptoms. However, it is important to note that eucalyptus oil should not be ingested as it can be toxic (Salem, et al. 2023).

2. Elderberry (Sambucus nigra):

Elderberry is a well-known immune-boosting herb, but it is also beneficial for respiratory health. Elderberries contain anthocyanins that have anti-inflammatory and immune-modulating effects. Consuming elderberry syrup or tea can help relieve symptoms of respiratory infections, reduce congestion, and support the immune system. It is particularly effective in managing cold and flu symptoms. However, it is important to note that elderberry should be used with caution in individuals with autoimmune disorders. Also, it is advisable to consult with a healthcare professional before consuming elderberry products, especially if you are taking immunosuppressive medications.

3. Mullein (Verbascum thapsus):

Mullein has been utilized for centuries to treat respiratory conditions due to its expectorant and soothing properties. It can help ease coughs, clear congestion, and reduce inflammation in the respiratory tract. The leaves of mullein are often used to make tea or herbal infusions that can be consumed several times a day to alleviate respiratory issues. Additionally, mullein can be found in the form of tinctures or lozenges to provide targeted relief. Mullein is considered safe for most individuals, but pregnant and breastfeeding individuals should avoid using it due to limited research.

4. Licorice Root (Glycyrrhiza glabra):

Licorice root has long been recognized for its soothing and anti-inflammatory properties. It can provide relief from coughs, bronchial spasms, and respiratory infections. Licorice root is available in various forms such as tea, capsules, and lozenges. The compound glycyrrhizin in licorice root has been found to increase mucosal secretion and reduce cough severity. However, it is essential to use licorice root cautiously, as excessive consumption may lead to high blood pressure. It is not recommended for individuals with hypertension, kidney disease, or hormonal disorders. Long-term use or high doses of licorice root should also be avoided.

5. Thyme (Thymus vulgaris):

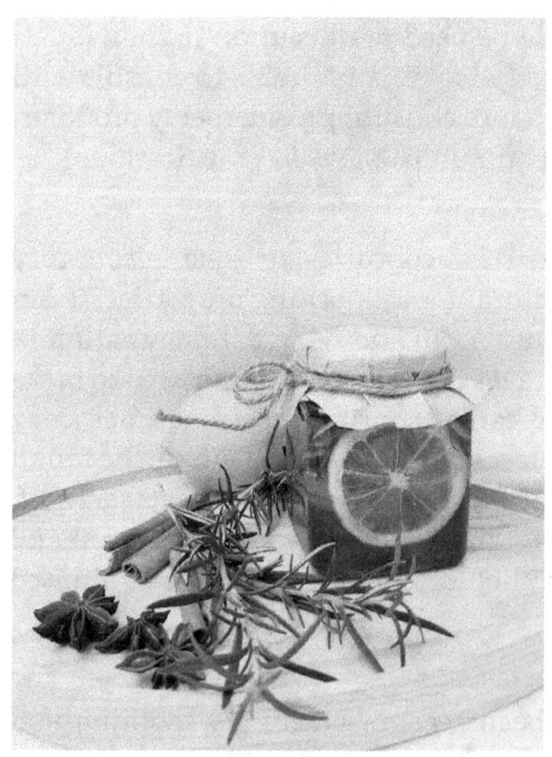

Thyme is a potent herb with exceptional antimicrobial and expectorant properties. It can help alleviate respiratory infections, bronchitis, and congestion. Thyme tea, made from leaves or dried thyme, can be consumed regularly to promote respiratory health. Additionally, thyme essential oil can be used in steam inhalations for more immediate relief from respiratory symptoms. Thyme is also known to enhance the function of cilia, the tiny hair-like structures in our airways that help clear mucus and debris. However, individuals with a history of allergic reactions to thyme or other members of the Lamiaceae family should exercise caution when using thyme.

6. Osha Root (Ligusticum porteri):

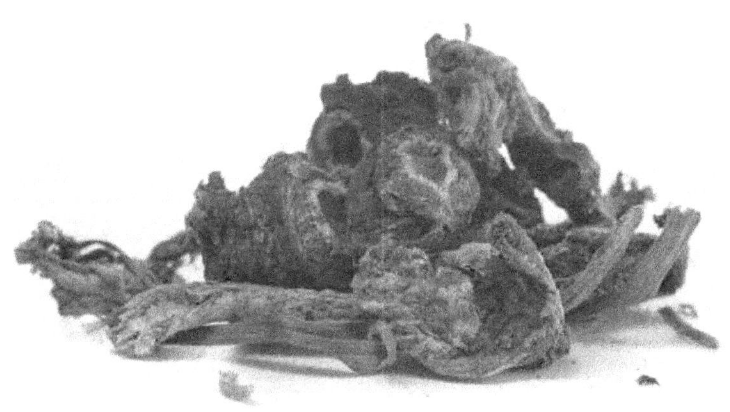

Osha root is a powerful herb native to the high-altitude regions of North America. It is known for its ability to support respiratory health and alleviate respiratory congestion. Osha root acts as an expectorant, helping to clear mucus buildup in the lungs and bronchial tubes. It also has antiviral and antibacterial properties that make it effective in fighting respiratory infections. Osha root is often used in the form of tinctures or capsules and should be used under the guidance of a healthcare professional. Individuals with bleeding disorders or those taking blood-thinning medications should avoid using osha root.

7. Coltsfoot (Tussilago farfara):

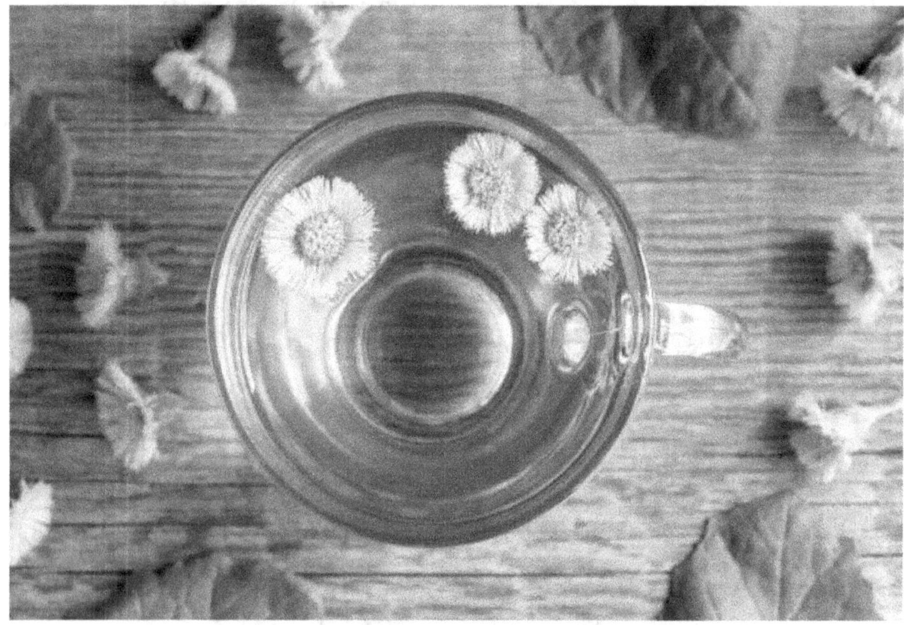

Coltsfoot has been used for centuries to ease coughs, bronchial congestion, and asthma. The leaves of the Coltsfoot plant contain mucilage and compounds that help soothe the respiratory system. Coltsfoot can be consumed as a tea or used in herbal formulations to alleviate respiratory symptoms. It is important to note, however, that Coltsfoot should not be used over an extended period or by individuals with pre-existing liver conditions. Pregnant individuals should also avoid using Coltsfoot due to its potential for liver toxicity. Always consult with a healthcare professional before using Coltsfoot or any other herbal remedy, especially if you have underlying health conditions.

It is important to consult with a healthcare professional or herbalist before incorporating herbal remedies into your respiratory health regimen, especially if you are currently taking any medications or have underlying medical conditions. While herbal remedies can be highly effective, it is crucial to find the right combination and dosage for your specific needs.

Remember, respiratory health is crucial for leading a fulfilling and active life. By incorporating these herbal remedies into your daily routine, you can support your respiratory system and breathe freely once again.

CHAPTER 14
Herbal Remedies for Pain Relief

Pain, whether acute or chronic, can be a distressing experience that hampers our daily activities and overall well-being. While modern medicine provides various pharmaceutical options for pain management, many individuals are turning to herbal remedies as a natural alternative. The use of herbs for pain relief dates back thousands of years, and their efficacy and safety have stood the test of time. In this chapter, we will delve deeper into the world of herbal remedies, exploring a range of plants renowned for their analgesic and anti-inflammatory properties, and offering effective and sustainable solutions for pain relief.

1. Turmeric (Curcuma longa):

Known for its vibrant yellow color and distinct flavor in curry dishes, turmeric has been used for centuries in traditional Ayurvedic and Chinese medicine. The active compound in turmeric, curcumin, possesses potent anti-inflammatory properties that inhibit the production of inflammatory enzymes, providing relief from conditions such as arthritis, joint pain, and muscle soreness. Additionally, curcumin acts as a natural pain reliever by influencing pain pathways in the body. Turmeric can be consumed in various forms, including fresh root, powder, or as a supplement. To enhance its absorption, it is often paired with black pepper, which contains piperine, a compound that enhances curcumin's bioavailability.

2. Willow Bark (Salix spp.):

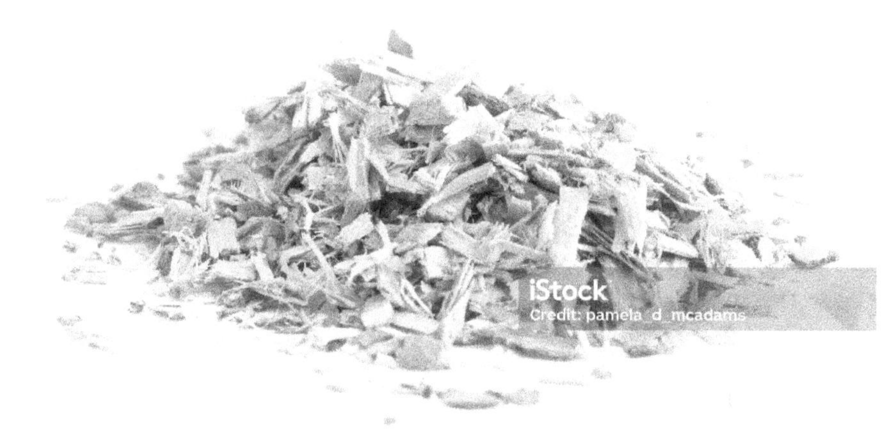

Willow bark has been long recognized as a natural pain reliever. The bark of various species, such as white willow (Salix alba) and black willow (Salix nigra), contains salicin, a compound that is like aspirin in its chemical structure and provides pain-relieving and anti-inflammatory effects. Willow bark has been historically used to alleviate headaches, back pain, and osteoarthritis discomfort. It can be brewed into tea or taken as a supplement.

However, those with salicylate sensitivities or who are taking blood-thinning medications should exercise caution when using willow bark.

3. Devil's Claw (Harpagophytum procumbens):

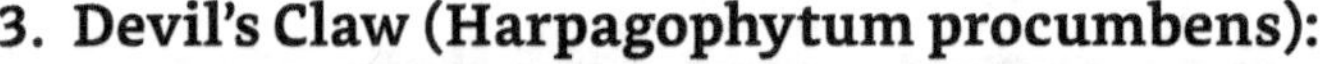

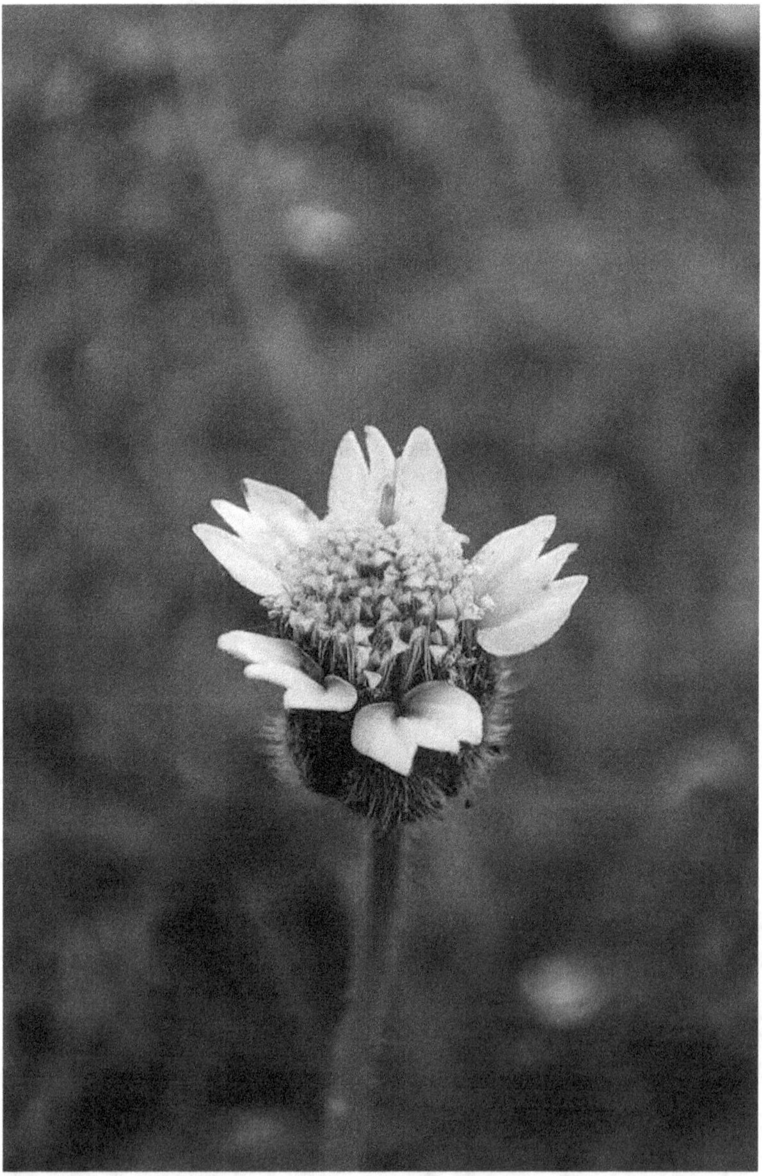

Native to the arid regions of southern Africa, devil's claw has a long-standing reputation for managing chronic pain. Its tuberous roots contain harpagosides, which possess anti-inflammatory and analgesic properties. Devil's claw is particularly effective in reducing pain associated with conditions like arthritis and lower back pain. It can be consumed in capsule or tea form or applied topically as a poultice to relieve joint and muscle pain. Some studies have suggested that devil's claw may also have potential benefits for reducing the use of nonsteroidal anti-inflammatory drugs (NSAIDs) due to its' effectiveness.

4. White Willow Bark (Salix alba):

White willow bark, derived from the white willow tree, has been used since ancient times as a natural analgesic and anti-inflammatory agent. With high salicin content, it offers pain relief by inhibiting the production of prostaglandins, which contribute to pain and inflammation. This herb has been employed to alleviate symptoms of conditions such as migraines, menstrual cramps, and joint pain. It can be consumed as a tea or taken in capsule form. However, individuals with salicylate allergies, asthma, or who are taking certain medications should avoid white willow bark.

5. Jamaican Dogwood (Piscidia erythrina):

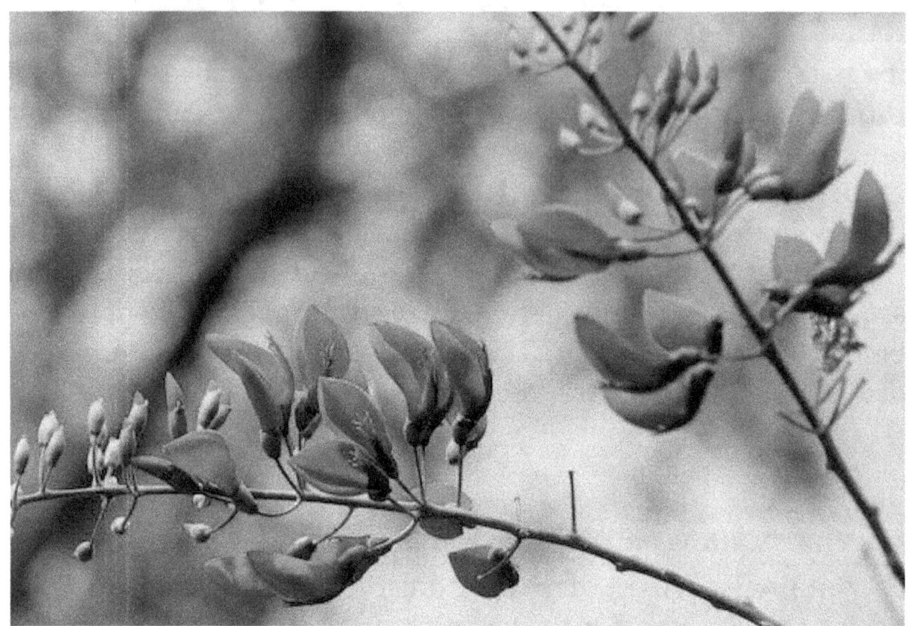

Native to the West Indies, Jamaican dogwood has a long history of use in traditional medicine for its potent analgesic properties. It contains compounds such as alkaloids and flavonoids that act as natural pain relievers and sedatives. Jamaican dogwood is particularly effective in nerve pain management, including conditions like neuralgia, migraines, and toothaches. This herb is commonly consumed as a tincture or in capsule form. Due to its sedative effects, it is advisable not to drive or operate heavy machinery after its use. It also has muscle-relaxing effects, which may contribute to its pain-relieving properties.

6. Arnica (Arnica montana):

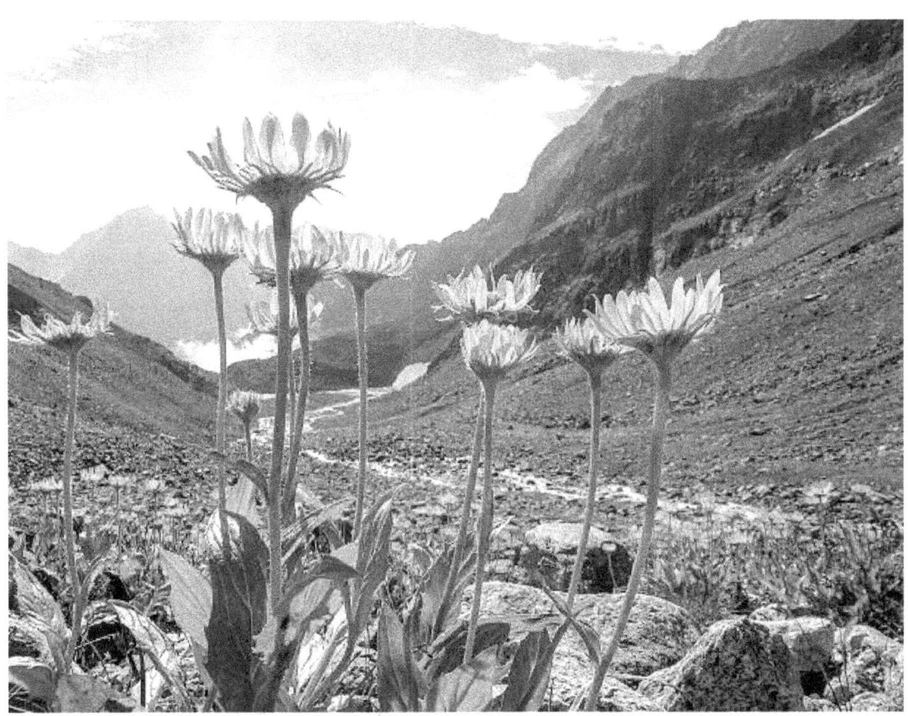

Arnica, a sunflower family member, is a popular herb used topically for pain relief and reduction of inflammation associated with bruises, sprains, and muscle soreness. Its active compounds, such as helenalin and flavonoids, possess anti-inflammatory properties that promote healing and alleviate discomfort. Arnica can be applied as a cream, gel, or ointment to the affected area up to several times a day. However, it should not be used on broken skin or open wounds. Arnica has also been investigated for its potential benefits in reducing postoperative pain and inflammation.

7. Meadowsweet (Filipendula ulmaria):

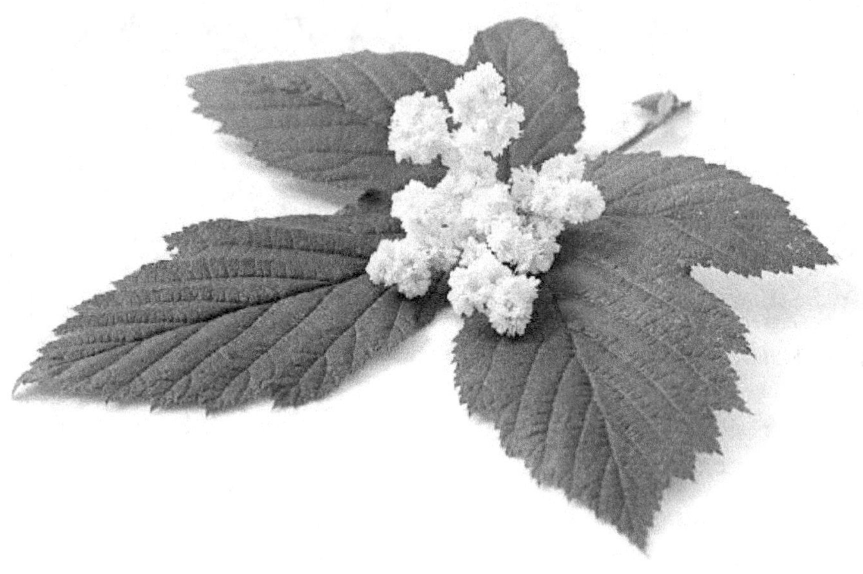

Meadowsweet, also known as "queen of the meadow," has a rich history of use in traditional European medicine. It contains salicylates that are converted to salicylic acid in the body, known for their pain-relieving properties. Meadowsweet has been commonly used to alleviate symptoms of conditions such as headaches, migraines, and general pain. It can be consumed as tea or taken in capsule form. Individuals with salicylate sensitivities or who are taking medications that interact with aspirin should exercise caution when using meadowsweet.

8. Clove (Syzygium aromaticum):

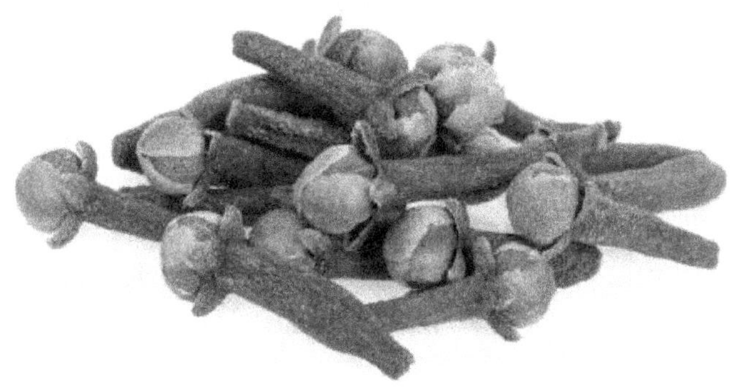

Clove, derived from an evergreen tree, is a well-known spice often associated with dental pain relief, but its benefits extend beyond that. The active compound in cloves, eugenol, exhibits both analgesic and anti-inflammatory properties. Clove oil, which contains high concentrations of eugenol, can be applied topically to relieve toothaches, sore gums, and temporomandibular joint (TMJ) pain. It can also be used as a mouth rinse for oral pain relief. Additionally, cloves can be consumed in the form of tea, adding a warming and soothing element to pain relief.

When incorporating herbal remedies into your pain management routine, it is crucial to approach them with caution and consult with a healthcare professional beforehand, especially if you have pre-existing health conditions, taking medications, or are pregnant or breastfeeding. Although herbal remedies are generally safe, they may have potential side effects or interactions with certain medications. Remember to start with low doses, monitor your body's response, and discontinue use if any adverse reactions occur.

In conclusion, herbal remedies offer a natural and often effective alternative for pain relief. By harnessing the healing power of plants, we can manage pain in a holistic and sustainable way, helping us live more comfortably and enjoy life to the fullest. Whether you choose turmeric, willow bark, devil's claw, white willow bark, Jamaican dogwood, arnica, meadowsweet, or clove, incorporating these herbs into your pain management regimen can provide relief and enhance your overall well-being.

CHAPTER 15
Herbal Remedies for Sleep and Relaxation

A good night's sleep is not only a luxury; it is an absolute necessity for our physical and mental well-being. Unfortunately, in today's fast-paced world, many people struggle with occasional or chronic insomnia, restlessness, and difficulty in achieving deep and restorative sleep. Thankfully, nature has blessed us with a wide array of herbal remedies that have been traditionally used to promote relaxation and improve sleep quality. In this chapter, we will delve deeper into these medicinal plants and explore their unique properties (Burns, 2023).

1. **Chamomile (Matricaria chamomilla):**

With its dainty, daisy-like flowers, chamomile is a herb that has been revered for centuries as a sleep aid and for its calming effects. This gentle sedative is rich in compounds called flavonoids, which have anti-anxiety and mild sedative properties. Chamomile is known to calm the nervous system, alleviate anxiety, and induce sleep. As a popular choice before bedtime, chamomile tea is a sweet and comforting infusion that helps relax the mind and body. But beyond its sleep-inducing effects, chamomile also offers other benefits. It has been found to possess anti-inflammatory properties, aid digestion, and soothe menstrual cramps. Additionally, chamomile can be applied topically to soothe skin irritations, such as eczema or rashes.

2. Valerian (Valeriana officinalis):

Valerian root, with its earthy aroma and potent sedative properties, is a powerhouse herb when it comes to improving sleep quality and reducing anxiety. This ancient remedy works by increasing the levels of gamma-aminobutyric acid (GABA) in the brain, a neurotransmitter that inhibits the transmission of nerve impulses, thus promoting relaxation and calmness. Valerian is commonly used to treat insomnia and has been shown to improve sleep latency, depth, and overall sleep quality. Research suggests that Valerian may also help reduce symptoms of restlessness, nervousness, and stress. However, it's important to note that Valerian may cause drowsiness, it's advisable to avoid activities that require alertness, such as driving, after taking it.

3. Passionflower (Passiflora incarnata):

The delicate and vibrant passionflower not only delights the eyes but also possesses remarkable relaxation-inducing properties. This beautiful herb has been used for centuries to alleviate insomnia and anxiety. Passionflower is believed to work by increasing GABA levels in the brain, thus reducing stress, and promoting restful sleep. Various studies have shown that passionflower can reduce sleep disturbances and improve sleep quality. Additionally, passionflower has been found to possess anxiolytic effects, making it beneficial for reducing anxiety levels and inducing a sense of tranquility. Some research suggests that passionflower may even enhance the efficacy of prescription sleep medications, allowing for lower dosage requirements.

4. Lavender (Lavandula angustifolia):

Lavender, with its heavenly scent and calming effects, is a beloved herb in the realm of relaxation and sleep. Its aromatic compounds have been shown to reduce anxiety and promote relaxation by interacting with neurotransmitters in the brain. Incorporating lavender into your bedtime routine can have profound effects on sleep quality. In addition to diffusing lavender essential oil or adding it to a bath, you can also consider using lavender-infused products, such as linen sprays or sleep masks, to enhance the relaxation experience. Lavender's benefits extend beyond sleep as well. It is commonly used for reducing stress levels, soothing headaches, and relieving muscle tension. Some studies have even suggested that inhaling lavender before bed can increase deep sleep and promote feeling refreshed upon awakening.

5. Lemon Balm (Melissa officinalis):

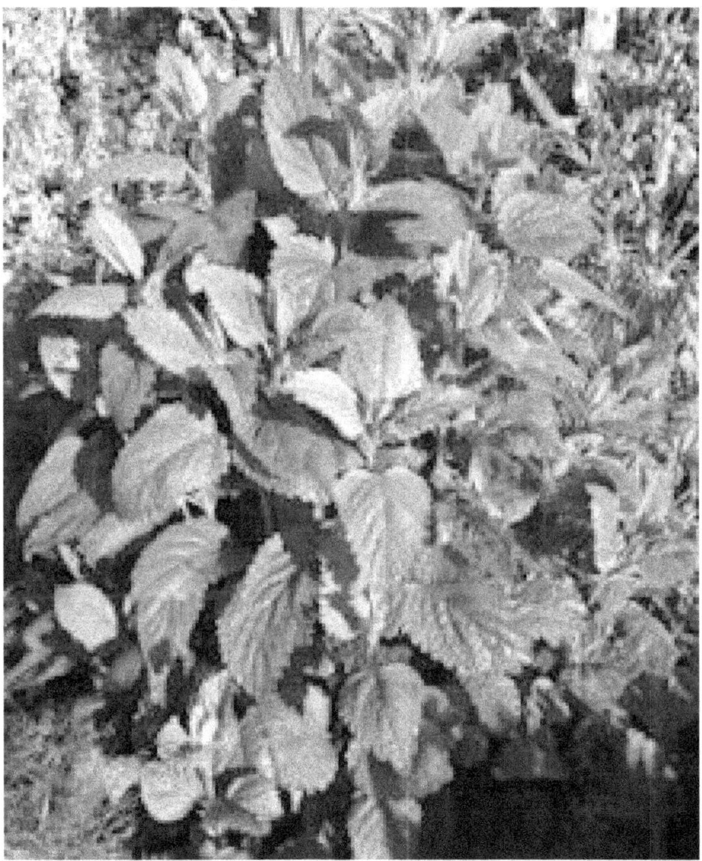

Known for its lemony fragrance and soothing properties, lemon balm is a gentle herb with calming effects on the nervous system. It has been used since ancient times to alleviate insomnia, restlessness, and anxiety. Lemon balm contains compounds that increase GABA levels in the brain, promoting relaxation and reducing stress. Research has shown lemon balm to be beneficial for improving sleep quality, reducing sleep disorders in children, and even alleviating symptoms of mild to moderate Alzheimer's disease. Additionally, lemon balm has demonstrated antiviral properties, making it a potential remedy for cold sores caused by herpes simplex virus.

6. California Poppy (Eschscholzia californica):

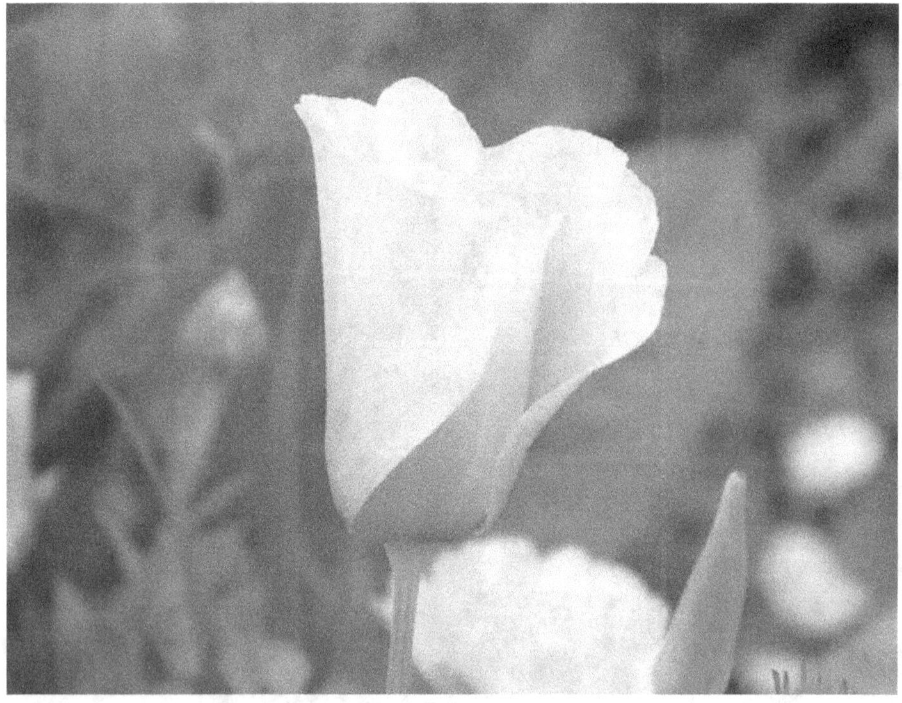

Originating from the sunny meadows of California, the vibrant orange blossoms of the California poppy hold immense medicinal value for those seeking better sleep. This gentle sedative herb has been used for centuries by indigenous cultures to promote relaxation and alleviate insomnia and nervousness. Research suggests that California poppy can improve sleep quality by reducing the time it takes to fall asleep and increasing overall sleep time. In addition to its sleep-inducing effects, California poppy also offers other benefits. It has been found to possess analgesic properties, aiding in the relief of pain and muscle spasms. This herb is also known for its gentle mood-enhancing abilities, providing relaxation without causing drowsiness.

While herbal remedies offer great potential for promoting sleep and relaxation, it's important to note that they may affect individuals differently. Before incorporating any new herbs into your routine, it is advisable to consult with a healthcare professional, especially if you have any underlying health conditions or are taking medications.

In addition to incorporating herbal remedies, practicing good sleep hygiene is vital for improving sleep quality. It's beneficial to maintain a regular sleep schedule, avoid electronic devices before bed, create a calm and peaceful sleep environment, and engage in relaxation techniques such as meditation or gentle stretching. By combining herbal remedies with these healthy sleep habits, you can enhance relaxation, promote restful sleep, and wake up feeling rejuvenated and ready to conquer the day ahead. Remember, finding the right combination of herbs and practices may require a bit of experimentation, so be patient, listen to your body's needs, and enjoy the journey to a more peaceful sleep.

Reference:

Abdulidha, N.A., Jacob, A.A. & AL-Moziel, M.S.G. (2020). Protective effects of Co-Q10, Ginkgo biloba, and L-carnitine on brain, kidney, liver, and endocrine system against sub-acute heavy metals toxicity in male rats. Toxicol. Environ. Health Sci.12, 331–341 https://doi.org/10.1007/s13530-020-00061-7

Burns J. (2023). Common herbs for stress: The science and strategy of a botanical medicine approach to self-care. Journal of interprofessional education & practice, 30, 100592. https://doi.org/10.1016/j.xjep.2022.100592

Calixto, J.B., (2005).Twenty-five years of research on medicinal plants in Latin America: A personal view. Journal of Ethnopharmacology, (100),1–2. pg131-134. ISSN

Demirbolat, I., Ulusoy, S., Inal, E., & Kartal, M. (2023). Variations in essential oil compositions and biological activities of Artemisia annua L. (sweet wormwood) at different growth periods. *Journal of Essential Oil Bearing Plants* (26)4, pages 10081017.

Dietz, B. M., Hajirahimkhan, A., Dunlap, T. L., & Bolton, J.L. (2016). Botanicals and Their Bioactive Phytochemicals for Women's Health. Pharmacological reviews, 68(4), 1026–1073. https://doi.org/10.1124/pr.115.010843

Ekor M. (2014). The growing use of herbal medicines: issues relating to adverse reactions and challenges in monitoring safety. Frontiers in pharmacology, 4, 177. https://doi.org/10.3389/fphar.2013.00177 https://files.nccih.nih.gov/files/licorice-root-steven-foster-square.jpg

Martin, F. , Michael, H. , Anthony, B. (2020). Medicinal Plant Analysis: A Historical and Regional Discussion of Emergent Complex Techniques. Frontiers in Pharmacology. (10). URL= https://www.frontiersin.org/journals/pharmacology/articles/10.3389/fphar. DOI=10.3389/fphar.2019.01480

Maja, D.C., Saller, R.,Leonti, M., & Weckerle,C.S. (2023)."Trends of Medicinal Plant over the Last 2000 Years in Central Europe" Plants (12)1,135. https://doi.org/10.3390/plants120101 35

Rubegeta, E., Ahmad, A., Kamatou, G. P. P., Sandasi, M., Sommerlatte, H., Viljoen, A.M. (2018). Headspace analysis, antimicrobial and anti-quorum sensing activities of seven selected African Commiphora species. South Afr. J. Bot. 122, 522–528. doi: 10.1016/j.sajb.2018.03.001

Saleem, M., Shaheen, M.A., Qadir, R.,Saba, I., Rehman, M.M., Paracha, R.N., Ahmad, N., Riaz, M. & Anwar, F., (2023) Variations in the composition and biochemical attributes of Eucalyptus camaldulensis L. leaves essential oil as function of drying methods. *Journal of Essential Oil Bearing Plants*(26)5,pages12661277.

Shawarb, N., Badrasawi, M., Qaoud, H. A., & Hussein, F. (2023). An ethnobotanical study of medicinal plants used for the management of respiratory tract disorders in northern parts of Palestine. BMCcomplementarymedicineandtherapies,23(1),387. https://doi.org/10.1186/s12906-023-04176-5

Welz, A.N., Emberger-Klein, A. & Menrad, K. (2018). Why people use herbal medicine: insights Use from a focus-group study in Germany. BMCComplementAlternMed18,92https://doi.org/10.1186/s12906-018-2160-6

https://www.fs.usda.gov/wildflowers/ethnobotany/medicina l/

index.shtml

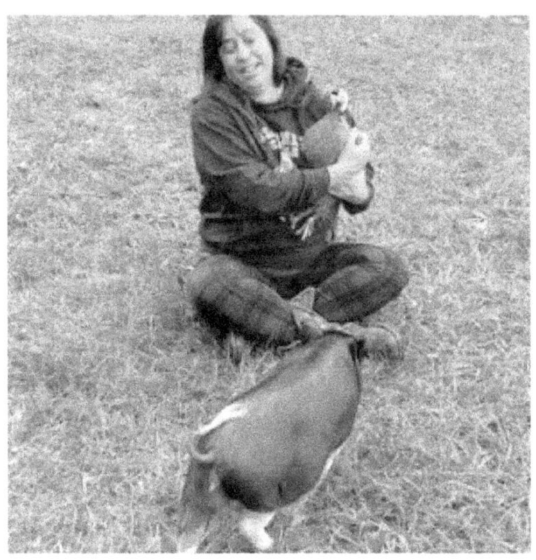

ABOUT THE AUTHOR

Catherine Sienna, a multi-talented individual, can be described as an extraordinary author, nurse, loving mother, and doting grandmother. Growing up, Catherine discovered the power and wonder that books hold, allowing her to escape into countless captivating worlds. This love for literature has become one of her life's greatest passions, a passion she eagerly shares with her children and grandchildren.

With a compassionate heart and an unwavering commitment to helping others, Catherine pursued a career in nursing. Her calling led her to specialize in mental health, where she provides essential care to those in need. Through her tireless dedication, Catherine strives to bring healing and support to individuals who are often overlooked or misunderstood, promoting overall well-being and emotional resilience.

You can connect with me on:

https://read.amazon.com/kp/embed?asin=B0CQW8YR2F&preview=newtab&linkCode=kpe&ref_=cm_sw_r_kb_dp_P2WSFFG2Q2QFE4T1AM0J

https://l.facebook.com/l.php?u=https://www.amazon.com/author/catherinesienna?fbclid=IwAR3gUVLDraueNPFyLHCfR0_SaaxIGqxiaWjJdRhWcun5OOT_HlV5LP2llU0&h=AT0S_3A7Y1422gE4dkqa6mQZAwImSB7nwkHOjafcymLsXaB2yAXMBibxMHXsXrIA9VFwaaoQ642F3pJuL3F0mUaDKjot8QGz0lLiav9

ALSO BY CATHERINE SIENNA

Catherine Sienna

AFTER 50

Becoming YOur Best
Self

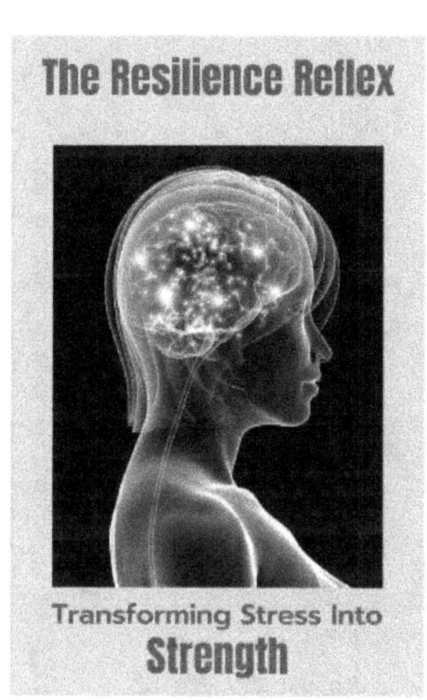